SO-DZG-623

'82

ASPIRATION BIOPSY FOR THE COMMUNITY HOSPITAL

David B. Kaminsky, M.D.

Director of Laboratories
Eisenhower Medical Center
Rancho Mirage, California

MASSON Publishing USA, Inc.
New York • Paris • Barcelona • Milan • Mexico City • Rio de Janeiro

Library of Congress Cataloging in Publication Data

Kaminsky, David B.
 Aspiration biopsy.

 (Masson monographs in diagnostic cytopathology ;
v. 2)
 Bibliography: p.
 Includes index.
 1. Tumors—Biopsy, Needle.   2. Diagnosis,
Cytologic.   3. Biopsy, Needle.   I. Title.   II. Series.
[DNLM: 1. Biopsy, Needle.   2. Hospitals, Community.
W1 MA9309RN v. 2 / WB 379 K15a]
RC270.K28   616.07'58   81-11720
ISBN 0-89352-154-X   AACR2

Copyright © 1981, by Masson Publishing USA, Inc.

All rights reserved. No part of this book may be reproduced in any form, by photostat, microform,
retrieval system, or any other means, without the prior written permission of the publisher.

ISBN 0-89352-154-X
Library of Congress Catalog Card Number: 81-11720

Printed in the United States of America

Masson Monographs in Diagnostic Cytopathology

Series Editor: William W. Johnston, M.D.

1. *Diagnostic Respiratory Cytopathology*

By William W. Johnston, M.D.
and
William J. Frable, M.D. (1979)

2. *Aspiration Biopsy for the Community Hospital*

By David B. Kaminsky, M.D. (1981)

DEDICATION

To Janice Kaminsky

and

To Joel H. Thayer, M.D.

for their exquisite friendship

Preface

The aspiration biopsy is about to experience a utilization renaissance in American medical practice. The renewal is justifiable, essential, and defies historical reluctance for its assimilation. A skeptical medical community repudiated Martin's initial introduction of fine needle aspiration cytology 50 years ago. His concept was avant-garde but perceptive, clairvoyant, and emphatically predictive. Avoidance of needle aspiration cytology as a diagnostic procedure was a reflective expression of the conservatism of the time: Frozen section diagnosis was evolving and exfoliative cytology was ingenue.

The technique was provocative, but only a select coterie of university pathologists was competent to judge malignancy from cell patterns transferred by needle from controversial lesions to glass rectangles. Unavailability of confident interpreters justified clinicians' hesitation, and translation was deferred to frozen section analysis, which offered the comfort of familiarity and a common vocabulary predicated on histoarchitecture. American laboratory medicine indulged in abdictation of its responsibility to develop expertise in the aspiration biopsy. A few centers transcended the skepticism and ambivalence and protected the procedure, but without active promulgation. The liberal Scandinavian attitude, objective and progressive, supervened and needle aspiration cytology became a European phenomenon. The exciting investigative and clinical work at Radiumhemmet by Franzen, Zajicek, and Esposti produced extraordinary results in breast and lung, salivary gland and thyroid, lymph nodes, and prostate, with corroborative biopsy data that verified that the criteria for cell diagnosis were faithful to tissue patterns and could be practically applied to clinical diagnosis of tumors without surgical intervention.

The milieu for the rejuvenation the aspiration biopsy in this country is an informed society with a significant tumor burden and correlative, escalating financial responsibility for its management. Needle aspiration cytology offers a versatile, precise, rapid, and cost-effective analytical method for primary or adjunctive diagnosis of oncological disease. Its adaptability as an outpatient procedure conserves costly hospitalization for biopsy and provides an alternative to exploratory incision. A cellular harvest may be acquired under direct vizualization, or by direction of fluoroscopy, computerized axial tomography, and ultrasonography. Availability of a diagnosis within 15 minutes of puncture permits the participation of the patient in the choice of therapy and in expediting the next stage of the therapeutic process.

The American Society of Cytology is committed to intensive national training programs designed to create confident pathologists who can disseminate the technique to the community hospital level where it achieves its vitality and viability. Frable, Hajdu, Melamed, Koss, and Kline have made exhaustive contributions to the evolution of the technique and have augmented the decentralization of patient care to the community.

This monograph is intended to testify to the applicability of fine needle aspiration cytology as an irrevocably essential procedure for patient care in the community hospital. It is designed to encourage utilization by presentation of cellular material that correlates cytoarchitectural features with tissue anatomy and clinical characteristics, emphasizing the necessity for close rapport between clinician and cytopathologist, and dynamic dialogue with the patient. It summarizes the gratifying early but developing experience of the author who introduced the technique to a sophisticated community hospital in which there was no prior exposure and celebrates the established confidence in the aspiration biopsy as an example of what is happening in this new and exciting era of cellular pathology.

Acknowledgments

This monograph was the conception of Professor William W. Johnston, the privilege of the author and the legacy of numerous individuals who share the vision that aspiration biopsy will prevail as a significant diagnostic modality. Dr. Johnston has been an inspiration because of his academic excellence and his enthusiastic desire to bring information about the cytologic method to students, cytotechnologists, and cytopathologists on a working, practical basis through his editorship of the Masson series in clinical cytology. I appreciate his influence and friendship. Dr. Jack Frable, who introduced me to the technique, has shared his wisdom and experience as mentor and friend. Linda Woolcox, CT (ASCP) has an incredible diagnostic acumen, an enviable talent for cytopreparation, and for continuous support in gathering and organizing the details of this book. Mathew Espinosa, the medical illustrator and photographer for the Eisenhower Medical Center, and William Boyarsky, his counterpart at Duke University, provided excellent photographic documentation and illustration for which I am grateful. The surgeons at Eisenhower Medical Center who accepted the technique on a trial basis, provided cases for study and eventually diagnosis, with ultimate belief in the procedure deserve gratitude: Dr. Joseph Lesser for the breast material, Dr. William R. Blakeley for lung, Dr. Stuart Barton and Dr. Robert Gebhart for thyroid, and Dr. Wayne Garrett for universal samples. The courage of the radiologists to use their equipment for directing the needle to its tissue targets is to be admired and appreciated. Dr. Joel H. Thayer inaugurated the radiological cooperation, believed the technique would be profitable for patients and for academic contribution, and encouraged its use. Dr. Richard Lynch has incredible talent for sampling minute lung lesions under fluoroscopy and Dr. Donald Wade for puncturing abdominal lesions visualized on CT scans magnificently prepared by Tom Tracia. Their contributions to this work are self-evident and immeasurable. I appreciate Dr. Stephen Hajdu's enthusiasm in initiating my interest in cytology and for continuing to maintain standards of excellence at the Memorial Hospital by which we endeavor to function in the community hospital. I am grateful to Lisa McFadden for preparation of the manuscript and to William Hoese, Laboratory Manager for the Eisenhower Medical Center for analysis of cost containment. I appreciate Dr. Connell Cowan's influence.

Several cases presented in the monograph represent hybrids of cytology with an x-ray, a tissue section with an aspirate, to amplify or illustrate the point with optimal clarity of example.

A special thanks is indicated for Mr. Alan Frankenfield for his supportive and cooperative posture in the publication the manuscript.

David B. Kaminsky, M.D.

Contents

1 Justifications

PHILOSOPHY

The physician who commits his professional practice to a community hospital environment confronts certain paradoxes. He implicitly accepts responsibility for the health care of the individuals who are permanent residents or transients within the community, and his involvement often requires emotional and philosophical support beyond the scope of diagnosis and therapy. Yet, he is restrained to functioning within the delineated context of its technical facilities, which are often limited by space, financial endowment, and location remote from university centers. Despite these restrictions, the community hospital is required to maintain commitment to excellence and sustained superior performance in meeting the burgeoning health care needs of the local population. The cancer burden and its financial ramifications have escalated to enormous proportions on the community level. Early diagnosis with open communication to the patient and cost containment are dominant in the perspective of community medicine. Bed space, operating room facilities, and therapy units are in desperate need of expansion but are curtailed by certificates of need. The burden of creative and imaginative utilization of existing advantages is projected back to the physician, and his personal role in directing a diagnostic maneuver, informing the patient of results, and accomplishing therapy is intensified. This is the milieu in which recrudescent interest in fine needle aspiration biopsy was stimulated.

There exists an unprecedented public con-sciousness about health, medicine, and cancer that has been encouraged by mass media, legislation, and the feminist movement. Awareness has eventuated in a demand for early diagnosis, informed consent for the diagnostic maneuver, and patient participation in the selection of therapy. The progressive physician can accommodate to this enlightened posture by offering aspiration biopsy as a vehicle to rapid, early diagnosis of cancer with conservation of costs, anxiety, and inconvenience. This may be accomplished in the context of existing facilities, which may be utilized more judiciously with release of coveted bed space and operating rooms.

The conventional protocol for evaluation of a palpable mass or radiographically detected lesion involves open biopsy, frozen section, and the preparation of time-consuming histological slides, which delay final diagnosis and the scheduling of therapy while perpetuating the anxiety of the unknown. Although there is considerable effort to accomplish this selectively on an outpatient basis, most visceral biopsies require hospitalization with utilization of bed space and operating room facilities that are at a premium in the community hospital. Incisive invasion often requires sustained hospitalization for recovery. The medical status of some individuals may preclude surgery for establishing a diagnosis of cancer, and the financial burden of hospitalization may be prohibitive for others. For those individuals who are surgical candidates for exploratory investigation, but whose lesions are strategically situated adjacent to vascular or deep structures that contraindicate scalpel intervention, an atraumatic technique for cellular sampling would be most advantageous. Finally, there are malignant lesions that are best managed by radiation therapy or combined systemic chemotherapy, and a procedure that obviates exploratory surgery would conserve morbidity and concomitantly provide a tissue-equivalent substitute on which therapy may be predicated.

Fine needle aspiration cytology is the revolutionary technique that satisfies these advantages. The implements are inexpensive and ubiquitous in hospitals, clinics, and private offices and consist of disposable 22-gauge needles, 20-cc syringes, 95% ethanol, glass slides, antiseptic solution, and optional local anesthetic. A palpable or radiographically demonstrable lesion is required if this analytical method is to be successful. Close rapport between the physician and cytopathologist with open dialogue directed at patient support and involvement is essential. The detailed technique of the aspiration biopsy is described in subsequent chapters and will not be reiterated here, but the processing and analysis can be accomplished within 10–15 minutes of puncture. This makes the procedure particularly applicable to first visit analysis in a clinic or private office, because a palpable lesion, for example in breast, lymph nodes, or soft tissues, can be aspirated and analyzed while the patient waits; the diagnosis can be related and the therapeutic plan formulated. The anxiety of the interval between biopsy and release of results is minimized. Patient comfort, support, and understanding of the disease process are amplified. The need for hospitalization, operating room time, and possible morbidity are eliminated for the diagnostic phase. If the patient presents a high medical risk that precludes surgical intervention, the placement of a needle by visual direction, fluoroscopic guidance, or computerized tomographic control is the atraumatic alternative for establishing the diagnosis. The needle may be used intraoperatively with great success to reach inaccessible lesions adjacent to vascular structures, or to biopsy the pancreas without threatening its fragility and precipitating pancreatitis. Thoracotomy may be obviated by acquiring a cellular sample from an undifferentiated lung carcinoma, "oat cell type." Aspiration of the thyroid may spare the patient a surgical procedure by providing cellular evidence of thyroiditis or evacuating the contents of a cyst. Metastatic dissemination of a known tumor can be substantiated and the cell type categorized to assist in the selection of suitable chemotherapeutic agents or to plan radiotherapy. If surgical extirpation of a lesion is the treatment of choice, preliminary diagnosis of cell type will direct an efficient operation by drafting the fields, scheduling block time, anesthetic support, and conserving the tissue of small lesions for sophisticated accessory studies, such as hormonal receptor assays, immunological markers, and cultures. If the suspicious lesion is an inflammatory process rather than a tumor, the needle is efficacious in selecting material for morphological identification of the specific agents of infection and for inoculating selective culture media.

There are limitations. The accuracy of diagnosis is variable with the experience, training, and technique of the cytopathologist and may be modulated by his relationship with the clinician, radiologist, and patient. The greatest accuracy is obtained when the interpretor of the cells also performs the puncture and assesses the clinical environment from which the sample is derived. In the series of the avid, experienced devotées of the technique, accuracy approximates 90%, and equivocal cases are referred for histopathological confirmation. The clinician is reminded that a negative aspiration result does not unequivocally exclude malignancy, particularly if there is a high clinical index of suspicion for cancer, and further intervention is requisite. A diagnosis of benignancy in the appropriate clinical context, however, provides a rational means for patient surveillance based on scientific merit. Certain inflammatory processes may imitate cancer with vicious mimicry and defy even the most capable cytodiagnostician, but even histological analysis is not without the atypia of reaction and repair, cellular subterfuge in the disguise of tissue. A secure sense of organ-specific criteria must pervade the consciousness of cytodiagnosis in this new media that does not always correspond to exfoliative cytology. Fine needle aspiration cytology cannot discriminate the subtleties of a process that requires exhaustive histological effort: follicular adenoma of the thyroid cannot be distinguished by this method from follicular carcinoma, which depends on thorough evaluation of the entire capsule and application of elastic stains to search for angioinvasion. Malignant lymphoma cannot be exquisitely subclassified or characterized as to its diffuse or nodular patterns, or B-cell, T-cell constituents, factors that impinge directly on treatment and prognosis. Despite these exceptions, the global application of the procedure should justify its implementation.

The medical community requires that the purveyors of this method are competent in its execution, that reliable diagnosis is the end result, and quality assurance is in effect. To this end, there are professionally sponsored courses and seminars that teach the technique, cytointerpretation, and clinical application. The literature is now an international forum with an overwhelming contribution of case reports, treatises, and monographs that explain the procedure, provide cellular criteria of diagnosis, technical suggestions, and report complications, caveats, and successful statistics. Quality control programs are amended to include needle aspirate specimens in the surveillance and testing systems. There is an urgency for the technique to disseminate, and time and circumstances are fertile for the community hospital to seize the moment.

COST CONTAINMENT

The improvement and ongoing monitoring of efficiency in the hospital in the delivery of health care is a formidable, but necessary task in view of current demands for both cost containment and high quality medical care. In the long run, effective cost containment depends on increased productivity. Wages and benefits represent approximately 60% of total hospital costs; therefore management of productivity of the physicians, nurses, and other technical staff will have the greatest impact on cost containment. With the current high interest in cost reduction and control, any technique that fosters these objectives should be thoroughly explored, and needle aspiration provides the advantage.

When a cost comparison of the needle aspirate versus the more conventional (surgical) technique is made, the most immediate and spectacular savings are seen in cases of nonmalignancy. Three cost studies that we conducted indicated that the needle aspiration biopsy can be performed at 10–30% the cost of the conventional hospital procedure. The cost of disposable supplies is negligible and the expenditure of pathologist's time is within reason.

Using average unit costs and a relative value system guide for services, we analyzed three common situations in which biopsy is a prelude to additional therapy or assures benignancy. We investigated the differences in cost between conventional biopsy and fine needle aspiration techniques. Table I summarizes the accounting for a conventional breast biopsy performed under anesthesia in the operating room of a community hospital contrasted with the charges for aspiration biopsy in the physician's office. The aspiration biopsy costs approximately 12% of the estimate for tissue biopsy. If the lesion is not malignant and the patient is dismissed, the savings exceeds 1100 dollars. If the conventional biopsy is malignant and results in modified radical mastectomy at the same sitting, the additive costs approximate 4300 dollars. If the aspirate is malignant and mastectomy is subsequently elected, a savings of 1100 dollars is preserved in the patient's behalf. Obviously, the most dramatic conservation of costs accompanies a benign situation.

In Table II the financial investment and predicted savings for needle aspiration of a thyroid cyst following confirmation by isotopic localization and ultrasonographic characterization is compared with lobectomy and frozen section. Both aspiration and conventional excisional biopsies are concomitantly therapeutic procedures for management of the cyst, and neither relies exclusively on preliminary radiographic techniques. The identification, evacuation, and cellular analysis by fine needle aspiration cytology costs in excess of 500 dollars, or 20% of the financial liability for lobectomy. If the lesion is not malignant, the savings involved exceeds 2200 dollars. The cost benefit is considerably diminished if the needle aspirate identifies malignancy and extended thyroid surgery is

TABLE I

Cost Differences Between Conventional and Aspiration Biopsy in Breast Cancer

Mastectomy—conventional			Mastectomy—needle aspirate		
Action	Unit Cost	Total Cost	Action	Unit Cost	Total Cost
Patient feels lump			Patient feels lump		
Physician visit (office)	$ 45.00	$ 45.00	Physician visit (office)	$ 45.00	$ 45.00
			Fine needle aspirate by pathologist	52.00	52.00
Hospital admission					
Laboratory					
Complete blood count	16.10		Materials		
Urinalysis	12.25		Slides (4)	.20	
VDRL	12.25		Jar alcohol (1)	.17	
Potassium	11.50	52.10	Syringe (20 cc)	.49	
			Needle (22 gauge)	.09	
Chest x-ray	45.60				
Electrocardiogram (over 40			Swab packet	.01	
years of age)	41.00	86.60	Sponge	.03	.99
1 day presurgical hospitalization at $178.00 per day	178.00	178.00	Pathology charges	48.00	48.00
Surgery			Total (nonmalignant)[a]		$145.99
Excisional biopsy (surgeon)	300.00				
Frozen section	66.00				
Tissue processing	49.50				
Pathologist consult	53.00				
Recovery room	100.00	568.50			
Anesthesiologist (30 min)	135.00				
Anesthesia mask	23.00	158.00			
Operating room (30 min) at					
$90.00 per 0.25 hr.	180.00	180.00			
Total (nonmalignant)[a]		$1,268.20			
If malignant:					
Operating room (60 min)	360.00				
Recovery room	100.00	460.00			
Laboratory charge	183.50	183.50			
Anesthesiologist (60 min)	270.00	270.00			
Surgeon's fee	1,200.00	1,200.00			
5 days postoperative hospitalization	890.00	890.00			
Subtotal		3,003.50			
Total		4,271.70			

[a]If non-malignant, savings is the difference between $1268.20 and $145.99, or $1122.20

indicated, but operative time is reduced and the necessity for frozen section may be eliminated, restraining accruing charges.

In Table III the cost factors in the identification of a lung tumor in a patient who presents with history of progressive cough is assessed. If the patient is admitted for conventional bronchoscopic biopsy in the operating room, and the results are benign, the cost is approximated at 1000 dollars in comparison to needle aspira-

tion biopsy under fluoroscopic guidance that costs half as much. If the bronchoscopic biopsy is inconclusive or malignant and lobectomy is pursued, the cost escalates to 6000 dollars. If the needle aspirate is positive for oat cell carcinoma, the patient is referred for radiotherapy and the diagnostic cost is restricted to 500 dollars; this pertains to a positive diagnosis of a nonresectable lesion. If a positive aspiration precedes lobectomy, the financial savings are inconsequential. In

TABLE II
Cost Difference Between Conventional and Aspiration Biopsy of Thyroid Cyst

Thyroid cyst—conventional			Thyroid cyst—needle aspirate		
Action	Unit cost	Total cost	Action	Unit cost	Total cost
Patient feels lump in throat			Patient feels lump in throat		
Physician visit (office)	$ 100.00	$ 100.00	Physician visit (office)	$100.00	$100.00
Thyroid scan-radioisotope (op)	215.75		Thyroid scan-radioisotope	215.75	
Ultrasound (op)	117.90	333.65	Ultrasound (op)	117.90	333.65
			Fine needle aspirate by pathologist	52.00	52.00
If positive					
Hospital admission					
Laboratory-Surgical Aids	100.75		Materials		
Electrocardiogram	41.00	141.75	Slides (4)	.20	
			Jar alcohol (1)	.17	
1 day presurgical hospitalization					
at $178.00 per day	178.00	178.00	Syringe (20 cc)	.49	
			Needle (22 gauge)	.09	
			Swab packet	.01	
Surgery			Sponge	.03	.99
Remove lobe for frozen section	1,343.00				
Frozen section	66.00		Pathology charges	48.00	48.00
Tissue processing	183.50				
Pathologist consult	53.00	1,645.50	Total (nonmalignant)[a]		$534.64
Anesthesiologist (30 min)	135.00				
Operating suite (30 min)	180.00	315.00			
Total (nonmalignant)[a]		$2,713.90			
If malignant:					
Additional surgeon's fee:	73.00				
Anesthesiologist	135.00				
Operating suite (30 min)	180.00	388.00			
Frozen section	66.00				
Tissue processing	183.50				
Pathologist consultation	53.00	302.50			
5 days postoperational hospitalization	890.00	890.00			
Subtotal		1,580.50			
Total		$4,294.40			

[a]If nonmalignant, saving is the difference between $2,713.90 and $534.64 or $2,179.26

these instances, cost containment may in part be a function of histological type.

From the hospital's point of view, operating room time can be more effectively and efficiently scheduled and time can be found for other types of surgery that are now postponed, or in some cases never done. Also, in the community hospital where bed space is limited, keeping patients out of presurgical beds frees space for others who need it and who sometimes by necessity must be transferred to other institutions.

In addition, it can be postulated that not performing the biopsy frees the time of not only the operating room, but also of the surgeons, the anesthesiologists, the nurses, and, in the laboratory, the histotechnologists. Reducing the work load of the technologists can result in holding staffing levels down without a sacrifice in quality of patient care.

PSYCHOSOCIAL ADJUSTMENTS

The patient population we have served with aspiration biopsy is a mélange of culturally diverse individuals with unique but divergent educational status, sophistication, and philo-

TABLE III

Cost Difference Between Conventional and Aspiration Biopsy in Lung Cancer

Lung carcinoma—conventional			Lung carcinoma—needle aspirate		
Action	Unit cost	Total cost	Action	Unit cost	Total cost
Patient has cough			Patient has cough		
Physician visit (office)	$ 50.00	$ 50.00	Physician visit (office)	$ 50.00	$ 50.00
Chest x-ray	45.60	45.60	Chest x-ray	45.60	45.60
Admit for 1 day hospitaliza-					
tion bronchoscopy at			Fine needle aspirate by pa-		
$178.00 per day	$ 178.00	$ 178.00	thologist	52.00	52.00
Laboratory			Admit 1 day hospitalization	$178.00	$178.00
Help panel	116.00				
Coag panel	42.00		Materials		
Complete blood count	16.10		Slides (4)	.20	
Urinalysis	12.25	186.35	Jar alcohol (1)	.17	
			Syringe (20 cc)	.49	
Surgical biopsy	100.00		Needle (22 gauge)	.09	
Frozen section	66.00		Swab packet	.01	
Tissue processing	49.50		Sponge	.03	.99
Pathologist consultation	53.00	286.50			
			Pathology charges	48.00	48.00
Operating suite	180.00				
Anesthesiologist	135.00		Radiology fee	150.00	150.00
Anesthesia mask	23.00	338.00			
Total (nonmalignant)[a]		1,084.45	Total (nonmalignant)[a]		524.59
If malignant:					
Surgical fee	2,200.00				
Blood	166.00				
Operating suite (60 min)	360.00				
Anesthesiologist	270.00	2,996.00			
Frozen section	66.00				
Tissue processing	183.50				
Pathologist consultation	53.00	302.50			
Postoperative hospitaliza-					
tion 10 days	1,780.00	1,780.00			
Subtotal		5,078.50			
Total		$6,162.95			

[a]If malignant, patient goes for radiation therapy. If nonmalignant, savings is the difference between $1066.45 and $524.59, or $541.86

sophical capability, subtending a spectrum from young adult to senior citizen. Yet it is unified by its vulnerability to cancer, by the unexpected penumbra cast by the sudden occurrence of a mass, cyst, or x-ray shadow that could irrevocably alter or extinguish life. Despite other differences, this unique population, suddenly and anxiously at risk, demands in unison to know immediately "Is it cancer?" Aspiration biopsy can provide the answer within 10 minutes of puncture.

The availability of a fast, reliable, atraumatic tissue-equivalent diagnostic method translates to a mechanism for informing the patient of his diagnosis at the premiere clinic or office visit. This pre-empts the crescendo of anxiety and fear that erupts during the interval between detection, the scheduling of hospitalization, performing conventional biopsy, and awaiting the histopathological results. If the biopsy is benign, and there is substantial clinical evidence that a surveillance program is reasonable, the patient is relieved of his concern. If the aspirate is malignant, confrontation with this information is immediate, and so is initiation of the physician's alliance in the coping process. There is a universal need for psychological adjustment to the burden of tumor with its implications for therapy, prognosis, and even planning for death. Early knowledge of the cancer diagnosis sets in motion the necessary dynamics of interpersonal adjustments for family and close friends.

There are practical reasons why patients want to be informed of their diagnosis early. The new consciousness and the feminist movement have created an awareness that the individual has jurisdiction over his body and that it is appropriate for him to participate in the choice of therapy for his cancer. Educated women prefer to discuss the alternatives to mastectomy, rather than awake from anesthesia to discover that this has been decided in their behalf. The aspirate diagnosis of cancer on an outpatient basis provides the opportunity for preliminary arrangements for child care during hospitalization, transportation to a radiotherapy facility or chemotherapist for sequential visits, and the ordering of legal affairs. Emotional inflammation imposed by financial burden may be partly ameliorated by the cost-containment advantages of early outpatient diagnosis in a setting that does not accrue daily hospital charges. The availability of the technique may encourage diagnosis in a patient who has resisted conventional biopsy because of fear of disfigurement or pain.

Our experience with fine needle aspiration cytology has been perpetuated in part because of patient request resulting from favorable reports on a lay basis within the community. There is interpersonal communication that a lump was detected, aspirated at the first office visit, a diagnosis rendered, and anxiety of waiting reduced or eliminated. Patients appreciate this more comfortable and informed approach to what otherwise could be a frightening medical experience. Aspiration biopsy is the vehicle to efficient diagnosis in a context that considers the patient's feelings and his emotional relationship to the diagnostic-therapeutic process.

MORBIDITY AND RISKS

The resurgent interest in fine needle aspiration biopsy has been promoted by the infrequency of complications it inflicts and by the minimal attendent morbidity. When carefully scrutinized, most allegations of complication are related to large-bore Vim-Silverman and other types of cutting needles and not to the 22-gauge instrument of cellular aspiration. Infection from the needle probe is rarely implicated or mentioned, but pneumothorax, hemorrhage, air embolism, and dissemination of tumor cells along the needle tract are given specific reference. A statistical approach to the validity of these complications is explicated in specific chapters, but in general there have been no significantly untoward results of the procedure in the extensive experience of Martin and Ellis,[1] Stewart,[2] Frable,[3] Hajdu and Melamed,[4] Kline and Neal,[5] and Zajicek.[6] Pneumothorax is virtually to be expected, is often asymptomatic with spontaneous resorption and pulmonary reinflation, and when clinically significant is manageable with insertion of a chest tube. Air embolism is infrequent because of the small diameter of the needle. Bleeding from the puncture wound is evanescent when it occurs, often controlled by pressure, and generally of minimal proportions as hemoptysis following lung biopsy. Translocation of tumor cells along the needle tract is only anecdotally documented,[7] representing an occurrence of perhaps one in many thousand cases, usually in association with a highly malignant tumor that can be predicted to have spontaneously disseminated widely. If the contraindications to specific organ puncture are respected and conventional technique is used, the complications are clinically inconsequential.

REFERENCES

1. Martin, H. E., and Ellis, E. B.: Biopsy by needle puncture and aspiration. *Ann Surg* **92**: 169–181, 1930.
2. Stewart, F. W.: The diagnosis of tumors by aspiration. *Am J Pathol* **9**: 801–812, 1933.
3. Frable, W. J.: Thin-needle aspiration biopsy. *Am J Clin Pathol* **65**(2): 168–182, 1976.
4. Hajdu, S. I., and Melamed, M. R.: The diagnostic value of aspiration smears. *Am J Clin Pathol* **59**(3): 350–356, 1973.
5. Kline, T. S., and Neal, H. S.: Needle aspiration biopsy: a critical appraisal. *J A M A* **239**(1): 36–39, 1978.
6. Zajicek, J.: Aspiration biopsy cytology I. Cytology of supradiaphragmatic organs. *Monogr Clin Cytol* **4**: 1–211, 1974.
7. Ferrucci, J. T., Wittenberg, J., Margolies, M. N., and Carey, R. W.: Malignant seeding of the tract after thin-needle aspiration biopsy. *Radiology* **130**: 345–346, 1979.

2 Getting Started

The decision to inaugurate fine needle aspiration cytology as a service modality to the medical staff is the cytopathologist's prerogative, but the program can be successful only if there is clinician acceptance and participation. This requires that the pathologist conveys a posture of confident self-assurance about his competence to render a cytological diagnosis on which definitive therapy may be predicated without confirmatory interim biopsy. Such self-assurance, as with other character traits, must be acquired through *process,* a dynamic experience of trial, cybernetic modulation, error, achievement, regression, progress. It must be communicated to recruit clinician support for utilization, treatment, and referral.

There are two phases in the implementation process: development of a collage of data points of reference concerning the characteristics and relationships of cells to their parent tissues of origin in normal, inflamed, and neoplastic structures, and convincing the clinician that these are reliable, if not preferred substitutes for the familiar, conventional, comfortable analytical methods to which he has become conditioned.

THE SURGICAL SPECIMEN LIBRARY: CELLULAR ACQUISITION FROM CONTROLLED ENVIRONMENTS

The luxuriant resource of the analytical data points resides in the surgical pathology material of the standard community hospital tissue laboratory.

The initial experience with fine needle aspirations depends on the intuitive utilization of unpreserved surgical specimens as the donor source of cells for structural studies, to imprint cellular patterns of recognition, and to stimulate associative cognizance of their relationship to histoarchitecture and gross features. A needle aspirate prepared from a mastectomy specimen is the introduction to the cellular aspects of breast carcinoma, and the synchronous preparation of the permanent histological slide expedites availability of familiar tissue for cross-comparisons. At the same time, it executes a permanent record of the malignant cells represented in the cytological milieu so that a subsequent recurrence in lymph nodes, chest wall, or lung may be sampled by clinical aspiration and compared in the same medium, to establish identity and proclaim metastatic progression. Creative exploration of surgical specimens that may have become routine or mundane confers an exciting perspective that rejuvenates interest in specimen analysis.

The pathologist who is a novice at the interpretation of needle aspirates must diligently and academically create a library of slides that compares the aspirated cells to corresponding tissue preparations using Papanicolaou's and hematoxylin-eosin stains fundamentally, and a flamboyant array of special stains to emphasize the myriad reactions and characteristics that cells maintain, even when disengaged from tissue congeries. The study sets should be carefully catalogued with organization according to disease process or organ source and retained in the cytology suite for accessibility. A duplicate slide of malignant lesions should be accessioned with the surgical pathology number and retained in the permanent file with the histological slides for comparison to subsequent clinical aspirates.

TECHNIQUE

Fine needle aspiration is appropriately termed because the needle utilized conventionally is 22 gauge and the material obtained is generally in a liquid medium, often almost invisible. This is in contradistinction to "needle biopsy," in which a needle perhaps four times the diameter harvests a solid core that is processed and evaluated as a histological preparation. Figure 2-1 dramatically demonstrates the small calibre of the 22-gauge needle in comparison to the common types of tissue biopsy needles. The penetration of the fine needle percutaneously for entry into a lesion requires a minute puncture wound (Fig. 2-2), for which local anesthesia is not requisite. The core biopsy needles are often introduced through a small incision by a scalpel blade after local preparation with Xylocaine. The needle tract produced by the 22-gauge probe is minute, inflicts minimal trauma, and avoids induction of

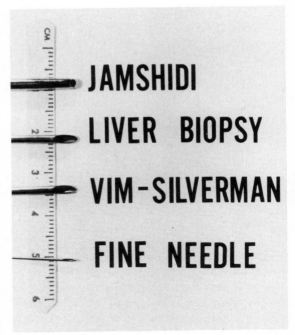

Fig. 2-1. Comparison of fine with conventional large bore biopsy needles.

bleeding. Figure 2-3 demonstrates the tract produced by a fine needle in a breast mass 4 days before, emphasizing minimal architectural disturbance. Although tumor cells diagnostic of

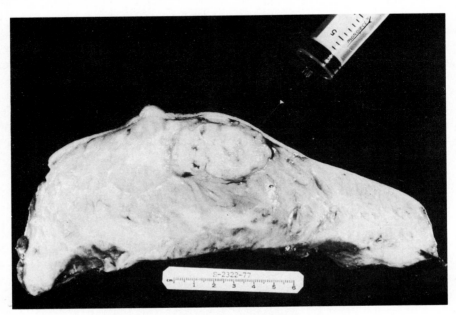

Fig. 2-2. Illustration of thin needle penetrating target.

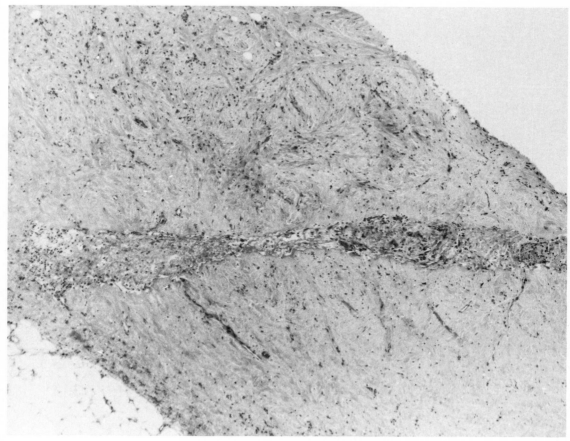

Fig. 2-3. Histological section, H&E, 62.5×, needle tract.

infiltrating lobular carcinoma were harvested, the cellular population of the tract lumen in this instance is a composite of inflammatory elements and fibroblasts responsible for repair (Fig. 2-4). Although it is recommended that the pathologist begin his specimen studies with a conventional 22-gauge needle available in his phlebotomy facility, it should be noted that clinical application with fluoroscopic or computerized axial tomographic (CAT) direction may require 22-gauge spinal needles to reach deep-seated lesions. Alternatively, the diagnosis of a benign colloid cyst of thyroid with secondary hemorrhage may require that a second puncture be performed utilizing an 18- or 20-gauge needle for evacuation of the blood decomposition products and colloid, to unite a therapeutic with a diagnostic effort. Accessible bone lesions are sometimes best approached with an 18-gauge

needle, but this selection comes spontaneously with experience. A pistol* is used for assisted facility in the aspiration procedure (Fig. 2-5).

A 20-cc syringe without Luer lock is best used to develop proper vacuum because cells must be displaced from their stromal support matrix by the action of aspiration, which implies and necessitates evacuation. Needle aspiration cytology differs from exfoliative cytology because in the former process cells are deliberately dislodged and displaced from tissue networks, whereas in an exfoliative harvest, this act is an indifferent and spontaneous ecdysiast disengagement of cells from stroma, an unprovoked uncou-

---

*The Cameco pistol is available through the Precision Dynamics Corporation, 3631 Thornton Avenue, Burbank, California 91504, and Aspir-gun is a product of The Everest Company, 5 Sherman Street, Linden, New Jersey 07036.

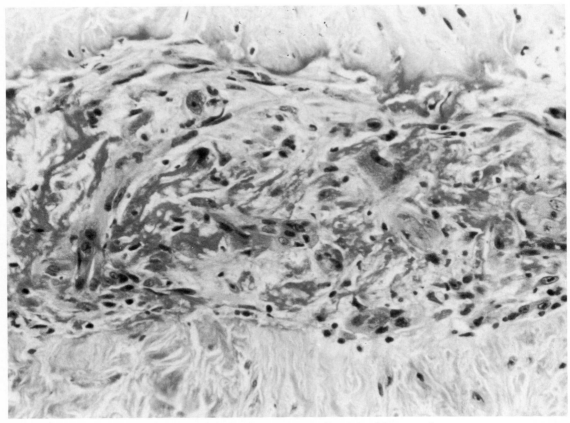

Fig. 2-4. Histological section, H&E, 400×, needle tract with reparative response.

pling. In our experience the 20-cc syringe is also a dexterous implement and may easily adapt to commercial syringe holders. In contradistinction to the European methodologies, we will evaluate only cytological material that has been meticulously fixed, preferably in 95% ethanol, with conscientious avoidance of artifact introduced by air drying. The Scandinavians developed their science of needle aspiration based on examination of cells with superimposed Romanowsky's stains after air contact exploded their cytoplasmic structure and denigrated nuclear detail. This approach provided an analytical product that was so disproportionately altered that correlation to tissue was severely compromised, and pathologists' incentive to attempt interpretation was harassed and discouraged.

Because optimal fixation is so germane to cellular preparation for clinical diagnosis, we insist on properly fixed specimens. Either the cytopathologist or cytotechnologist is present to assist the surgeon with specimen preparation to ensure proper handling. For those clinical cases aspirated by the pathologist, an assistant is always present to expedite fixation and smearing. Unfixed or air-dried specimens are automatically rejected as unsatisfactory. The discipline of fixation should commence during the period of learning from aspiration of surgical specimens, so that it becomes assimilated and automatic for the pathologist. The lid should be removed from the coplin jar containing 95% ethanol *before* the needle penetrates the tissue, so that the aspirator need not fumble with this activity while his cellular material shrivels on the drying slide.

An accessory fluid used in the procedure is normal saline, which need not be sterile. We complement our direct smears with a micropore filter preparation of a saline rinse of the needle. This provides additional material for study. In clinical application, such as fluoroscopically

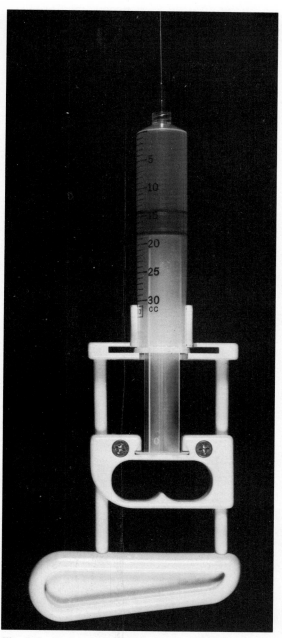

Fig. 2-5. Aspiration pistol for assisted facility in aspiration procedure.

TABLE I
Modified Papanicolaou's Stain

Filters:

1.	Ethyl alcohol	Minimum 15 minutes
2.	80% ethyl alcohol	10 dips
3.	70% ethyl alcohol	10 dips
4.	50% ethyl alcohol	10 dips
5.	Tap water	1 minute
6.	Gill's hematoxylin	2 minutes
7.	Tap water	Rinse until clear
8.	0.05% hydrochloric acid	Rinse filter until yellow
9.	Tap water	Rinse
10.	Scott's tap water	Rinse until filter appears to be blueing
11.	Tap water	Rinse
12.	50% ethyl alcohol	10 dips
13.	70% ethyl alcohol	10 dips
14.	80% ethyl alcohol	10 dips
15.	95% ethyl alcohol	1 minute
16.	Orange G stain	1½ minutes
17.	95% ethyl alcohol (3 dishes)	10 dips each
18.	EA stain	2 minutes
19.	95% ethyl alcohol (3 dishes)	10 dips each
20.	100% absolute isopropyl alcohol (2 dishes)	1 minute each
21.	Xylene	Minimum 10 minutes
22.	Coverslip	

redundant when the direct smear was unequivocally diagnostic.

We utilize the classical Papanicolaou's stain for the processing of cells aspirated from surgical specimens and from clinical cases for which an immediate response is not necessary (Table I). A modification of Papanicolaou's stain permits a rapid method that we use when an immediate assessment of specimen adequacy or the ultimate diagnosis is required. This occurs intraoperatively, or when radiological assistance, such as CAT scan direction is necessary and the patient must be retained in position on the procedure table until verification of sample or diagnosis is forthcoming. The classical and rapid modification of Papanicolaou's stain is included in Table II. Conformity to procedural detail will project a superb product.

Specimen aspiration, then, requires only fundamental equipment: a 22-gauge needle attached to a disposable 20-cc syringe, a coplin jar with 95% ethanol, a tube of normal saline,

directed aspiration of a pulmonary lesion, the saline wash may contribute additional material for acid-fast or fungal cultures. We have never regretted the extra few moments required to wash the needle, although admittedly, the accessory material may have been eliminated as

TABLE II
Modified Papanicolaou's Stain Method for Quick Stain of Aspiration Smears

95% ethyl alcohol	Minimum 3 minutes	95% ethyl alcohol	10 dips
70% ethyl alcohol	10 dips	95% ethyl alcohol	10 dips
Running tap water	5 dips	EA-50 stain	15 seconds
Gill II hematoxylin	30 seconds	95% ethyl alcohol	10 dips
Running tap water	5 dips	95% ethyl alcohol	10 dips
70% ethyl alcohol	10 dips	100% ethyl alcohol	10 dips
95% ethyl alcohol	10 dips	100% ethyl alcohol	10 dips
Orange G stain	15 seconds	Xylene	Minimum 30 seconds

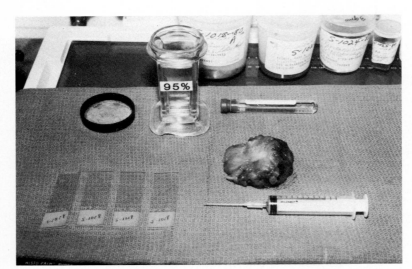

Fig. 2-6. Required implements for performing specimen aspirate.

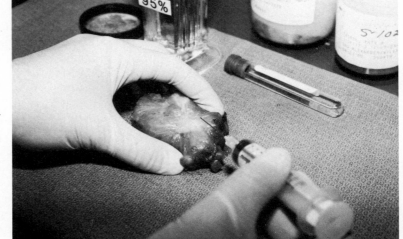

Fig. 2-7. The needle is introduced into the specimen.

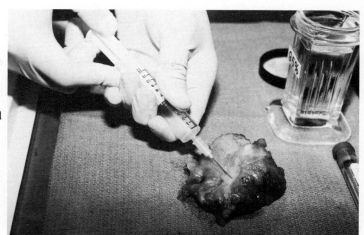

Fig. 2-8. The needle is repositioned while the vacuum is maintained.

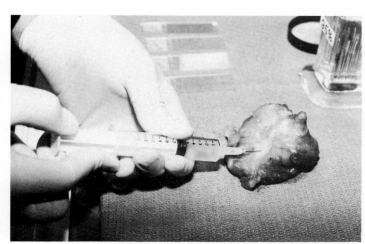

Fig. 2-9. Final repositioning of the needle prior to release of vacuum and withdrawal of specimen.

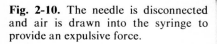

Fig. 2-10. The needle is disconnected and air is drawn into the syringe to provide an expulsive force.

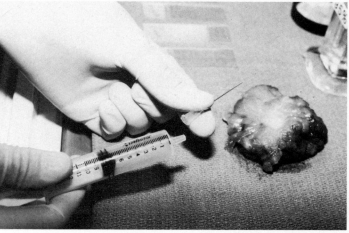

four glass slides, a fresh surgical specimen, and access to Papanicolaou's stain (Fig. 2-6).

The following procedural steps should be followed to perform a specimen aspirate:

1. Assemble the necessary equipment, label the slides, remove the lid from the coplin jar, and provide a clean work space.
2. Introduce the needle into the lesion (Fig. 2-7).
3. Withdraw the plunger of the syringe to create a vacuum (negative pressure), which will be transmitted to the interior of the tissue (Fig. 2-8).
4. Maintain the vacuum but reposition the needle by moving it in various directions to create a tissue cleavage plane into which the

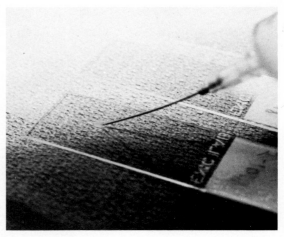

Fig. 2-11. The aspirated material is expressed onto the glass slides.

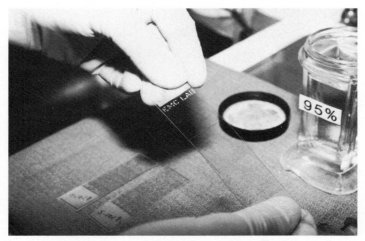

Fig. 2-12. The cellular material is dispersed in a circular monolayer.

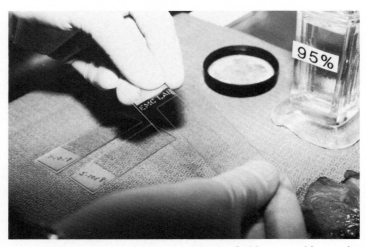

Fig. 2-13. The slides are separated in a perpendicular fashion to avoid smearing artifact.

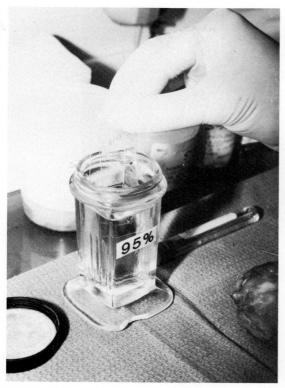

Fig. 2-14. The slides are immediately immersed in 95% ethanol.

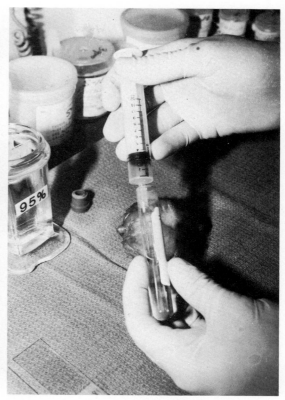

Fig. 2-15. A saline wash of the needle is prepared.

cells may be displaced for entry by vacuum into the core of the probing needle (Fig. 2-9). The action may be discontinued after four of five movements or if blood or other material appears at the hub of the syringe. It is important to avoid entry of the aspirated material into the barrel of the syringe because harvest is then difficult and cumbersome and considerable airdrying occurs as the material is transferred to slides.

5. Release the negative pressure before withdrawing the needle from the tissue. This prevents reflux of the material from the needle core into the barrel of the syringe.

6. After the needle has been withdrawn from the tissue, disconnect it from the syringe and fill the syringe with air to provide an expulsive force to eliminate the aspirated material from the interior of the needle (Fig. 2-10).

7. Reconnect the needle to the syringe and expel a droplet of aspirate on the end of the slide opposite the frosted square for label

application. This localizes the material for study and reduces screening area (Fig. 2-11).

8. Immediately touch the end of a second glass slide to the droplet and allow surface tension

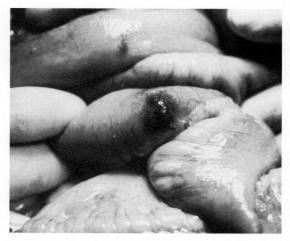

Fig. 2-16. Clinical photograph, small bowel at laparotomy with pigmented serosal lesion.

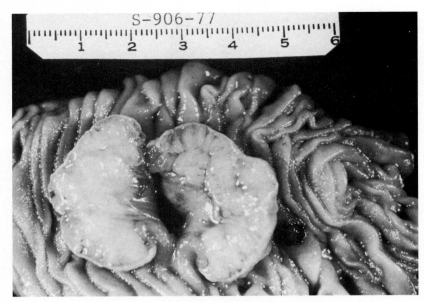

Fig. 2-17. Gross specimen, small bowel with submucosal metastatic malignant melanoma.

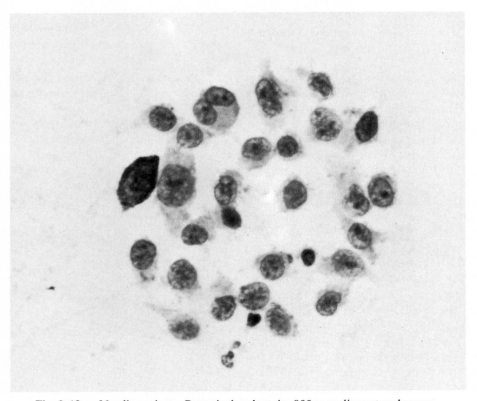

Fig. 2-18 a. Needle aspirate, Papanicolaou's stain, 800×, malignant melanoma.

to disperse the cells in a circular monolayer (Fig. 2-12). Separate the slides in a perpendicular dimension carefully avoiding the smearing action that is conventional for the preparation of peripheral blood smears (Fig. 2-13). This dispersal step is crucial because a thin layer is equivalent to proper fixation, acceptance of stain, and clarity of nuclear detail.

9. Immediately submerge both slides in the fixative and maintain for a minimum of 3–30 minutes (Fig. 2-14).
10. Aspirate normal saline into the barrel of the syringe and expel into the tube in repetitive sequence and then process the saline wash through a micropore filter or preserve for possible culture (Fig. 2-15).
11. Stain the material by Papanicolaou's technique or with accessory special stains to demonstrate such constituents as mucin, melanin, hemosiderin, hyaluronic acid.
12. Coverslip and label appropriately.

APPLICATION: SPECIMEN LIBRARY

In the early phases of developing expertise, the surgical specimen contributes the cells whose characteristics are learned from the visible gross and histoarchitectural features of a known quantity defined in familiar terms, on predetermined precepts. At a later time, this reverses, and cytoarchitecture becomes the reliable predicator of the nature of the surgical disease. The examples that follow are intended to provoke interest in applying the technique to specimen aspiration to acquire baseline information for later clinical decisions.

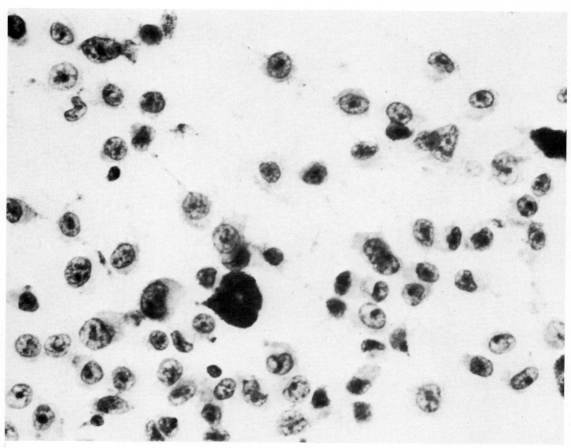

Fig. 2-18 b. Needle aspirate, Papanicolaou's stain, 800×, malignant melanoma.

Specimen Aspirate Number 1

A 53-year-old male was explored at laparo-tomy for decompression of bowel obstruction and identification of the source of intestinal bleeding. An intraoperative consultation was requested for the pathologist to evaluate pigmented, hemor-rhagic lesions violating the integrity of small bowel serosa (Fig. 2-16). A presumptive opinion of metastatic melanoma was expressed and segmental resection was accomplished. The mucosa of the small bowel segment was elevated by a subjacent polypoid mass with a lobulated, solid, nonpigmented interior that extended into muscularis propria with obliteration of submuco-sal tissues (Fig. 2-17). An adjacent, umbilicated, hemorrhagic, pigmented nodule ulcerated the mucosa.

A fine needle aspirate was selected from the polypoid excrescence (Fig. 2-18a) and stained by routine Papanicolaou's methods. The cellular population consisted of separately dispersed polyhedral cells with prominent, purple nucleoli, coarse chromatin dispersion, focal convolution-ary folding of nuclear envelopes and melanin pigmentation of the cytoplasm of some cells. These corresponded to sheeted aggregates of similar cellular units with cytoplasmic punctua-tion by finely stippled brown granules familiar to the surgical microscopist as melanin, as seen in a tissue section through the lesion (Fig. 2-19). The cellular features to be associated with malignant melanoma may be extrapolated from these comparisons, and except for the intranuclear vacuole, probably representing cytoplasmic in-vagination, which has been described in associa-tion with melanoma cells, the basic criteria can be deduced. It is unusual to find this artifact in needle aspirates, although it appears to be a reliable feature of spontaneously exfoliated

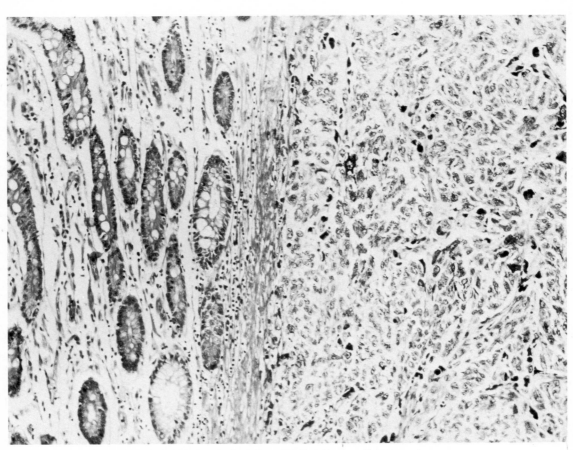

Fig. 2-19. Histological section, H&E, 160×, malignant melanoma.

melanoma cells, particularly in body cavity fluids. In some cells, melanin granules obscured the nuclei (Fig. 2-18 b). Careful reexamination of this patient's history revealed that a pigmented lesion had been excised from his back, but the practitioner who removed it elected to defer pathological examination of the tissue.

Specimen Aspirate Number 2

A 52-year-old male developed scalp nodules and was evaluated at another hospital where a biopsy was performed. A diagnosis of malignant tumor was made and he was referred to a surgeon at the Eisenhower Medical Center for wide excision. An irregular ellipse of skin and subcutis was excised under general anesthesia (Fig. 2-20) and the specimen was submitted in the fresh state (Fig. 2-21). The accessibility of the homogeneous, fleshy nodules to the surface is emphasized in the cross-sectional perspectives, suggesting that percutaneous aspiration could be easily accomplished (Fig. 2-22) clinically.

The aspirate was performed on the specimen according to the outlined technique and the dramatic cellular elements depicted in Figure 2-23 were obtained. The dominant cells were fusiform and straplike with longitudinal fibrils in the cytoplasm, bizarre multinucleation or lobation, thickened chromatin accentuating nuclear envelopes, prominent spiculated nucleoli, and tendency to fascicular adherence in small groups. Occasional cells had a polyhedral silhouette with an epithelioid suggestion. The corresponding histological sections (Fig. 2-24) demonstrated solid sheets of spindle, strap, and polyhedral cells, punctuated multifocally by individual cells with homogenized, eosinophilic, or granular cytoplasm with rudimentary cross striations. The tissue was considered representa-

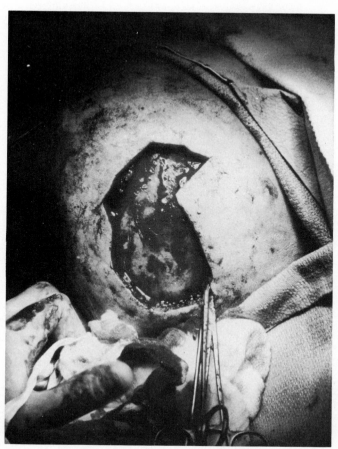

Fig. 2-20. Clinical photograph, scalp incision at surgery.

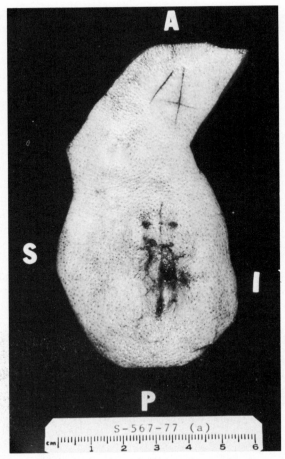

Fig. 2-21. Gross specimen, scalp incision incorporating multiple nodules of pleomorphic rhabdomyosarcoma.

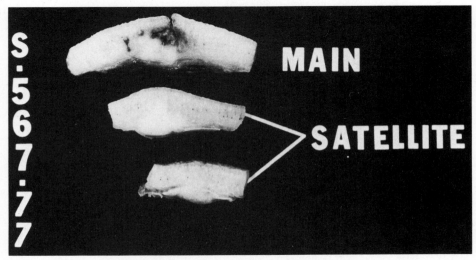

Fig. 2-22. Cross sections of scalp demonstrating proximity of lesion to surface and accessibility to needle probe.

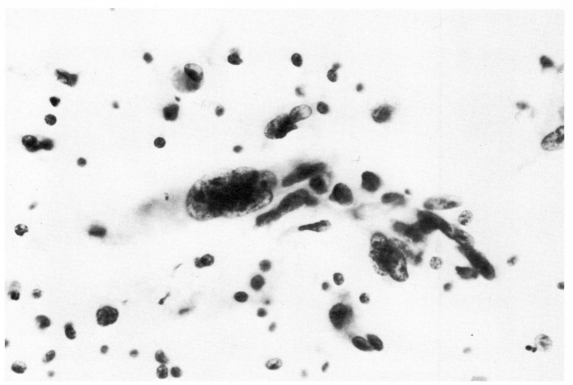

Fig. 2-23. Needle aspirate, Papanicolaou's stain, 625×, pleomorphic rhabdomyosarcoma.

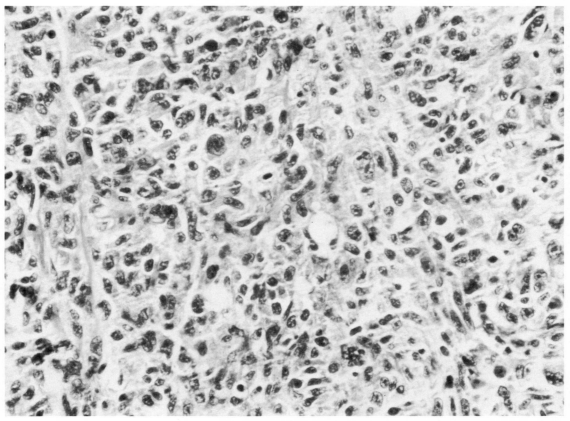

Fig. 2-24. Histological section, H&E, 400×, pleomorphic rhabdomyosarcoma.

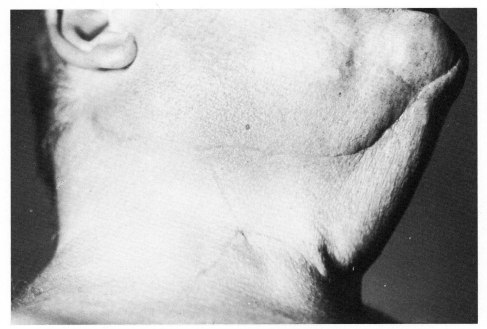

Fig. 2-25. Nodular recurrence in neck 1 year following radical neck dissection.

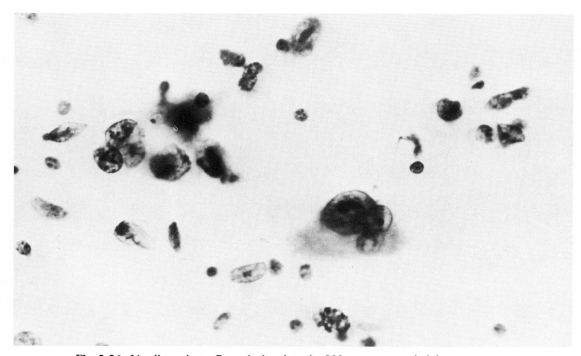

Fig. 2-26. Needle aspirate, Papanicolaou's stain, 800×, recurrent rhabdomyosarcoma.

tive of a pleomorphic rhabdomyosarcoma, and the features accentuated in the cellular preparation were recapitulated in organized tissue.

The postoperative course was uneventful and a subsequent radical neck dissection was done. A year later a nodular recurrence in the neck (Fig. 2-25) was evaluated by clinical aspiration and malignant cells identical with those in histological and previous specimen aspirates were found (Fig. 2-26). Since a specimen aspirate was available in the slide library for comparison with the clinical aspirate, identity was established. It was this case that prompted our conviction that all malignant tumors accessioned in surgical pathology should be sampled by aspiration to provide a baseline cytological example of the lesion for comparison with future clinical aspirates.

Specimen Aspirate Number 3

A 45-year-old active-duty military officer consulted a physician after experiencing acute onset of excruciating back pain after changing a

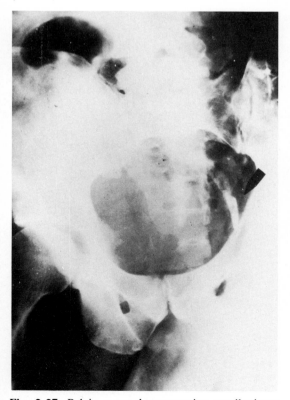

Fig. 2-27. Pelvic x-ray demonstrating cartilaginous mass.

TABLE III

Cellular Features of Chondrosarcoma by Specimen Aspirate Study of One Case

Cellular disportation	
Aggregation	97.7%
Single	2.3%
Nuclear shape	
Round or oval	78.7%
Reniform	21.3%
Multinucleation	0.3%
Mitoses	0%
Number of nucleoli/cell	
0	0.2%
1	71.1%
2	27.9%
3	0.8%
Nucleolar position	
Central	19.4%
Eccentric	80.6%

flat tire. Roentgenograms of the spine and subsequently the pelvis demonstrated a massive tumor projecting into the pelvis from the right sacroiliac junction (Fig. 2-27). A diagnosis of low-grade chondrosarcoma was established and a tumor committee recommended hemipelvectomy. The specimen provided an inexhaustible source of cells for study of this unusual lesion by fine needle aspiration cytology. The cells were therefore studied in the context of this diagnosis, and arbitrary parameters of cellular characteristics were assigned to a cytotechnology student* for extrapolation from his observation of approximately 2000 cells. These details are summarized in Table III and constitute the nucleus for accumulating knowledge of chondrosarcoma when it is represented cytologically.

By reviewing this information with the student, certain tentative observations could be defined for future modification, validation, and data bank entry. In this specimen, chondrosarcoma cells were communally aggregated into cohesive clusters with suggestion of cytoplasmic syncytial confluence (Fig. 2-28). Cells were rarely singly disported, but dehiscent elements carried with them a hint of lacunar demarcation (Fig. 2-29). Nuclei were predominantly round or oval, although reniform indentation of nuclear envelopes occurred in approximately 20% of the

---

*Appreciation to Wayne Recla, CT (ASCP) for this study.

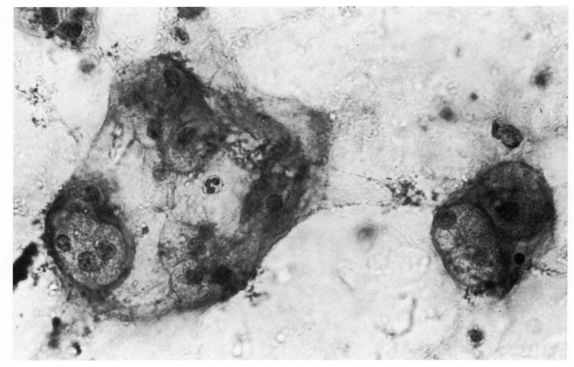

Fig. 2-28. Needle aspirate, Papanicolaou's stain, 600×, chondrosarcoma.

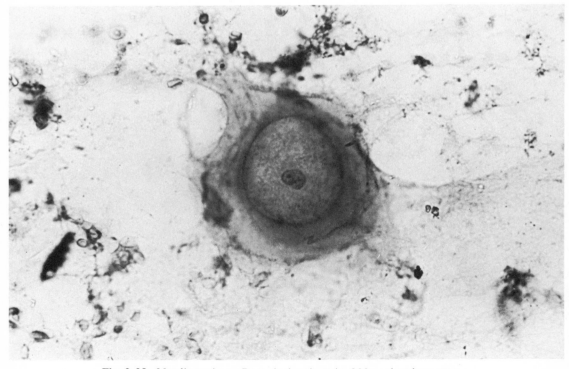

Fig. 2-29. Needle aspirate, Papanicolaou's stain, 800×, chondrosarcoma.

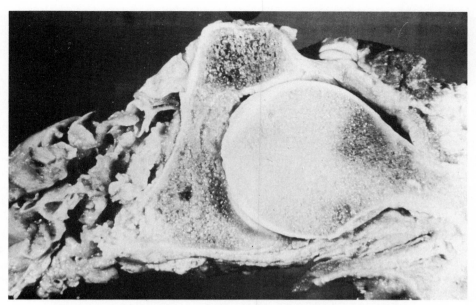

Fig. 2-30. Gross specimen, cartilaginous neoplasm destroying ilium.

cells. There were generally one to two nucleoli per cell with a predilection for eccentric displacement within the nuclei. Multinucleation and mitotic reduplication were essentially nonexistent. The malignant potential of the population subjected to analysis can be inferred from the destructive progression of tumor in the ilium adjacent to the femoral capital articulation (Fig. 2-30). The hypercellularity and crowding with disproportionate occupancy of chondroitin sulfate matrix, a familiar sign of cartilagenous malignancy to the surgical microscopist, characterized the histological sections (Fig. 2-31).

The inquisitive cytopathologist endeavoring to establish criteria leading to clinically useful applications and to the emergence of his credibility as a diagnostician by these methods must engage in exercises such as this. Questions of cell parameters, associations, morphological details that should be deliberately posed in the early experience of aspiration cytology later assume synaptic familiarity and become the disciples of the analyst probing cellular form to predict biological activity.

CONVINCING THE CLINICIAN: ENTRY INTO THE CLINICAL SPHERE

The second phase in the implementation of clinical fine needle aspiration is concerned with clinician consciousness about the reliability of the cytological diagnosis and cultivation of his trust in the approach. The pathologist needs to invoke his creativity as a diplomatic teacher to present a new perspective, reinforce its versatility, gently coerce the skeptic to acknowledge a new method, and by his intellectual integrity assure support, provide insight into the limitations, and above all sustain a high level of professional service to the consenting physician and his patient. If a diagnosis is equivocal, this must be communicated in precise terms, and professional conduct must survey ego-function. Consultation, an additional pass with the needle, or admission of inapplicability of the procedure for the specific case at hand can circumvent a regrettable and sometimes irrevocable diagnostic misjudgment. Pathologist familiarity with limitations of needle aspiration as a diagnostic tool must guide his consultative interaction with the clinical staff. For example, fine needle aspiration cannot precisely discriminate between a solitary follicular adenoma of the thyroid and an encapsulated low-grade follicular carcinoma, the distinction relying entirely on conscientious histological examination of the entire capsule of the lesion, using special stains to search for angioinvasion within its substance.

The campaign should be initiated with a well-constructed academic presentation of clinical aspiration to the medical staff at a formal grand rounds or mortality-morbidity conference. The format can parallel the approach of the didactic portion of workshops sponsored by the American Society of Cytology or American Society of Clinical Pathologists. At the initiation of our program, clinical material was limited from our own institution and we resorted to extramural examples and cases from the specimen aspirate file with radiological correlation when applicable. The scope of the presentation should be sufficiently versatile to titillate the interests of surgical subspecialists, radiologists, endocrinologists, and family practitioners, in addition to general surgeons and internists.

The surgeon's receptivity is enhanced by the willingness of the pathologist to appear in his office with a portable tray containing the equipment for the aspirate. The benefit of personal service by the pathologist is infinite. The surgeon's confidence to perform the mechanical aspirate is often supported by the pathologist who momentarily assumes a mentor role; the opportunity for observation of technique and recommendations for improvement is possible only through this corroborative effort of two consultants concerned with patient care. This posture ensures the pathologist's status as consultant (in the perspective of patient and surgeon) by affording him the opportunity of interviewing and examining the patient, engaging in dialogue that establishes rapport. The pathologist ascertains *for himself* the size, location, texture, and shape of the lesion that he must evaluate by its cellular envoys. For him this promotes accuracy of interpretation and avoids a depersonalized attitude toward the specimen, its source, and the problem. For the patient, there is reassurance that personal interest and combined effort are operative. The diagnosis is made available to the surgeon within 15 minutes while the patient is retained in his office. This rapid availability of diagnostic information allows patient participation in the choice and scheduling of

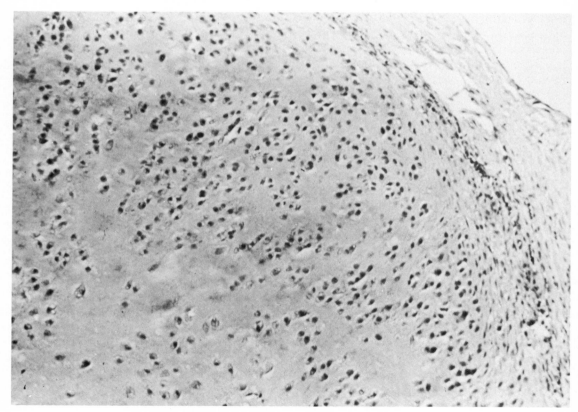

Fig. 2-31. Histological section, H&E, 160×, chondrosarcoma.

therapy, relieves the anxiety of the unknown, permits a second aspiration if the first specimen is inconclusive or if additional studies are indicated, and conserves a second visit that would otherwise be planned for discussion of the diagnosis.

The pathologist who advocates cytotechnologist integration in these diagnostic adventures further promotes the success of the program by developing an additional resource for assisting in specimen acquisition, particularly important for subsequent conflicts (in pathologists' time) that occur when concomitant aspirates are requested. Clinical exposure for the cytotechnologist improves his diagnostic performance and is tantamount to his recognition as a health professional in a system we must streamline by cost-effective, outpatient diagnostic endeavors.

The first clinical applications of fine needle aspiration at the Eisenhower Medical Center were interventions in the surgical breast service of private clinicians. The surgeons were receptive to doctrines promulgated through conferences and personal conversations of persuasion, but it was necessary to dispel skepticism with diagnostic accuracy. To achieve their confidence it was necessary in many situations to perform a fine needle aspirate, followed immediately by a parenchymal core biopsy with a conventional large-core diameter. The cytological specimen was processed and reported within 15 minutes, and the core was treated as a histological preparation with slides available within 24 hours. The concordance of diagnoses in most paired studies resulted in clinician acceptance of the aspirate method, and ultimately needle biopsy was abandoned. Bias in interpretation of the cytological specimen in the light of the tissue was precluded by the time interval, and the fine needle aspiration opinion was always rendered first. In most situations, however, the pathologist who interpreted the fine needle aspiration also interpreted the biopsy, but internal quality control review corroborated the findings. After the needle biopsy was disregarded in support of fine needle aspiration, a period of readjustment followed when frozen section confirmation of malignant cytological reports was requested before mastectomy or irradiation were accomplished. Confidence testing has now advanced fine needle aspi-

ration to the justifiable status of definitive diagnosis, and most surgeons proceed with mastectomy, sparing the time and cost of the frozen section, and conserving the tissue of small lesions for hormonal receptor assays.

Expansion of the diagnostic team to incorporate the radiologist is an intuitive act of unification that allows fine needle aspiration its greatest dimension, scope, and potential. The talented radiologist can creatively transform his knowledge of imaging and the abnormal silhouette to provide direction to the probing needle, advancing it to the precise position where an appropriate cellular harvest may be anticipated. For this effort, he extends facilities of fluoroscopy, CAT and ultrasonographic pattern displays to define the lesion and direct the needle. The pathoradiological force is a dynamic influence on patient care because the *directed* aspirate essentially assures a successful quantum of viable cells or organisms as a precise basis for further therapeutic or diagnostic intervention. Radionuclide imaging, particularly for thyroid nodules, invokes the participation of the radiologist committed to nuclear medicine.

Our radiological staff was inordinately receptive to their participation in fine needle aspiration as a reinforcement of the multidisciplinary approach to diagnosis. An educational process sponsored by the cytopathology staff was an essential preliminary preview of methodologies, expectations, limitations, and the mechanics of the cooperative approach. The cytopathologist or technologist provided assurance of his presence to assist with the preparation of all aspirates performed in the radiological suites. Diagnoses were delivered within 10 minutes and the patients could be retained on procedure tables until verification was assured. Work flow through the radiology department was expedited, and a satisfying attitude of contribution and academic achievement for patient welfare was formulated.

An anticipated problem that could develop in the context of community hospital-based physicians in a cooperative diagnostic effort is the threat to the clinician of his displacement from the primary diagnostic process. This did not occur at our institution because we embraced him as an equal partner, acknowledging his primary significance to the patient-doctor relationship, thereby diminishing any intrusive action our intervention might have predicated. The technique is now a viable, if not essential, component of our diagnostic armamentarium, and there are requests on certain days for as many as 10 fine needle aspirates, often concomitantly, in fluoroscopy, the CAT scan suite, private offices, and the special procedures room of the laboratory. We consider this a triumph in a 186-bed hospital where space and facilities are temporarily limited and the demand for action is overwhelming.

Finally, the modality of fine needle aspiration as an extension of diagnostic services from the anatomical pathology laboratory must be sustained within the jurisdiction of the cytopathologist. He has a responsibility for protagonist role in performing aspirates and conducting a clinical service for which he accepts referrals. This provides an alternative to the clinician who desires assistance or who may entirely abdicate the mechanics of cellular acquisition to his laboratory colleague. It is considerably more rewarding to the pathologist if he performs aspirates in addition to interpreting material submitted by other agencies.

The pathologist (and clinician) may commence clinical aspiration by extrapolating the identical technical methods from his practice with surgical specimens. He can elect to perform aspirates on deceased patients undergoing autopsy examination to assist with the transition from specimen to human subjects. The transfer of technique and method should be identical with the following exceptions. The patient is integrated into the process and must receive the following considerations: An explanation of the procedure in understandable language must lead to informed consent by discussing the mechanics of the puncture and aspiration, its diagnostic ramifications, and possible complexities of limitations or complications. The lesion must be stabilized, antiseptically prepared, and electively anesthetized. Evaluation must occur with urgency so that the sequence of fixation, stain, microscopy, report delivery can be efficiently executed.

Detailed photographic recapitulation of clinical methodologies will follow in the chapters on the fluoroscopically and CAT-scan directed biopsies.

Administrative considerations referable to hospital business must be introduced concomitantly. Fine needle aspiration should be a delineated privilege in the administrative documents of the Department of Pathology, with clarification of the training and experience, as well as continuing educational and quality control activities of the pathologists and cytotechnologist involved. A quality control program should be delineated and actively practiced and may include exchange of slides on an informal basis with local institutions or a respectable university center. Medical malpractice insurance generally covers this procedure if there is already provision for the pathologist to perform bone marrow aspirates and biopsies, but the procedure should be listed on applications for renewal and the carrier properly informed. Finally, a document that records the patient's acquiescence to the aspirate must be available, signed and witnessed as a formal expression of consent. The document may include a statement that information or photography can be used for purposes of continuing medical education, including publication.

CHAPTER 3

Aspiration Biopsy of the Palpable Breast Mass

The urgency provoked by the occurrence of a palpable breast mass has contributed immeasurably to the application and expansion of fine needle aspiration cytology as a diagnostic modality in this country. The majority of breast masses is initially detected by the woman or her lover, and there is an implicit, immediate spontaneous need to comprehend the significance of the mass and its consequences for the individual. The feminist movement has created an unprecedented consciousness about the body and promoted an intense awareness of corporal rights. Modern women want an immediate diagnosis of their breast lump and the opportunity to participate in the choice of therapy, particularly if the tumor is malignant. They no longer acquiesce to the perspective of learning about their cancers as they are revived from postmastectomy anesthetic somnolence but are conversant with the alternatives of "lumpectomy," radiation therapy, and simple mastectomy with prosthetic implantation. They actively invoke their rights to be informed and consulted about what is to happen to their bodies. Fine needle aspiration cytology makes it possible, and reliably realistic for their physicians to comply.

This procedure is designed to support an ambulatory, outpatient clinic or private office practice and permits in most instances of malignant disease an unequivocal diagnosis at the initial office visit, thereby reducing the psychological torment and anxiety that most women endure while awaiting processing of the conventional tissue biopsy. The cytological diagnosis is generally available within 10–15 minutes of the actual mechanical aspiration, and the physician is immediately informed so that he may relay the information to the patient. If a malignant diagnosis is ascertained, the therapeutic modalities are discussed and decided, and the patient has the opportunity to plan the details of hospitalization or sequential visits to a radiotherapy facility. A preoperative radionuclide and roentgenographic survey with laboratory testing may be initiated prior to hospitalization, so that the extent of malignant disease is substantiated and the surgical approach modified, if necessary.

The advantage to the surgeon is related to his scheduling of operative time, office patients, and postoperative visits. If modified radical mastectomy is the elected mode of therapy, the overwhelming trend at our institution is for the procedure to be done without interim confirmatory frozen section. This is not only a time- and cost-effective maneuver, but promotes conservation of small tumors for essential hormone receptor assays.

If the lesion is cytologically benign without atypia or proves to be cystic with an innocuous population of foam cells and apocrine elements, the patient may be assigned to a surveillance program to be re-evaluated at predetermined intervals. This may include repeat aspiration biopsy or mammography (Fig. 3-1). Mammography is inconsistently used in evaluation of the palpable mass, and its utilization varies with the philosophy, training, and experience of the clinician. In occasional cases, the mammogram may

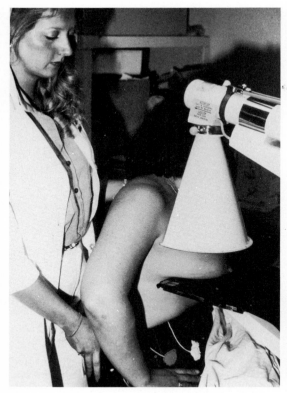

Fig. 3-1. Radiological technician prepares the breast for mammographic examination.

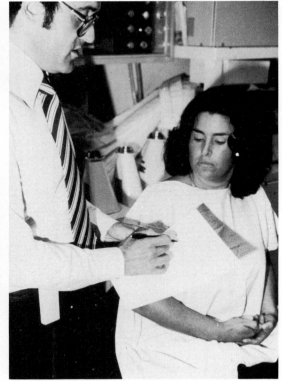

Fig. 3-2. The pathologist takes a history preparatory to performing the needle aspirate puncture.

serve to direct placement of the needle in a deep-seated lesion.

If the lesion is cytologically atypical or suspicious for malignancy, a recommendation for excisional biopsy and histological study is standard.

When the pathologist is consulted on a referral basis to evaluate the patient and perform the aspiration in addition to contributing the cytological interpretation, it is of paramount importance that he establish rapport with the patient, elicit a relevant history, and perform a physical examination of the breasts according to standard protocol (Fig. 3-2). The palpatory findings are significant for the clinical characterization and the localization of the lesion. Rimsten and associates[1] evaluated the diagnostic accuracy of clinical palpation and fine needle aspiration and their combined approach in the investigation of breast lesions and concluded that "a thorough palpatory evaluation is a prerequisite for a good result of aspiration biopsy, in particular to meet

the risk of a false negative cytological diagnosis." They evaluated 1244 women with breast symptoms by palpation and assigned their findings to a spectral category from "no cancer" to "cancer." Aspiration was performed in 984 breast lesions and the results were assigned to a category of "no cancer" through "slight, moderate and grave atypia" to "cancer." The correlated palpatory and cytological assignments achieved categorization of 91% of the proved cancers in the "cancer" to "strongly suspicious" palpatory group and the "cancer" to "grave atypia" cytological group.

The appearance of the aspirated material may correlate with the palpatory characteristics of the mass. Transparent greasy material may be consistent with lipid from adipose matrix or a lipoma, and the textural pliability and mobility of the gross lesion would correspond. An incompressibly indurated, fixed mass may be so desmoplastic that cells are not surrendered to the needle by tenacious fibrous frameworks, and the harvest may be unsuitable, requiring an additional pass. Necrotic material can indicate tumor, abscess, or fat necrosis and may prompt preparation of additional slides for special stains or extra samples for cultures. A fluctuant mass may be evacuated of its fluid content and residual tissue reassessed by an additional needle probe. Franzen and Zajicek[2] emphasized this correlative approach, relating the macroscopic appearance of the aspirate to the clinical problem and the cytoarchitecture. This was implicit in their conculsion that diagnostic accuracy increased proportionately when the cytopathologist who interpreted the slides also performed the aspirate. When the clinician is the vehicle responsible for the acquisition of the aspirate, it is preferable for the cytopathologist to be present to prepare the cellular material and witness the clinical interchange.

The spatial requirements for performing the aspiration biopsy are minimal and flexible. The standard treatment room in a clinical office or hospital floor affords comfort, privacy, and space, but certainly a segregated, private area of the phlebotomy section of the laboratory, a special procedures room, or the pathologist's office are acceptable. The aspirate may be done with the patient supine or sitting erect, and there is routinely no necessity for a postbiopsy recu-

perative period. Turn-around time can be minimal because the entire mechanical process requires only 5–10 minutes.

The aspiration is performed according to the principles delineated in Chapter 2. The mass is localized, immobilized, and the skin cleansed with an antiseptic. Local anesthesia is generally avoided. The lesion is perforated by a 22-gauge needle attached to a 20-cc syringe (Fig. 3-3). A vacuum is created by withdrawing the plunger of the syringe and the needle is repositioned variably to create tissue cleavage planes. The vacuum is re-equilibrated, the needle withdrawn, and the smears prepared, fixed, and stained according to conventional technique. The referring clinician is contacted by telephone and by a subsequent written document.

The pathologist who assumes responsibility for initiating fine needle aspiration biopsy as a routine and active diagnostic modality must analyze the risk involved in the procedure and conscientiously educate his clinical colleagues who provide the explanation and assurance culminating in informed consent. The immediate concerns invoked are those of hematoma formation, infection, and dissemination of tumor along the needle tract. In a more subtle perspective is the abstract problem of false negative and false positive diagnoses, which impact directly by

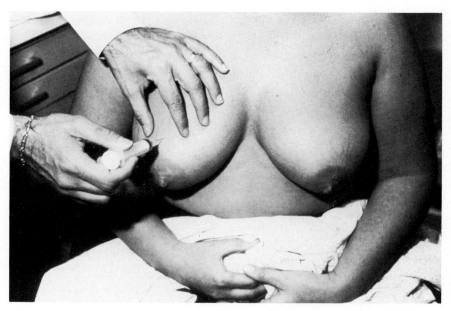

Fig. 3-3. The pathologist performs the puncture without accessory local anesthesia.

victimizing the patient through delaying therapy or overprescribing. A clear comprehension of these concerns will allow the process to proceed without anxiety or conflict. Kline and Neal[3] authoritatively stated that there is no known contraindication to the procedure. They are implicitly correct and our enlarging experience continues to justify this posture.

The most comprehensive experience with fine needle aspiration biopsy of the breast is a review of 3479 consecutive biopsies reported by Franzen and Zajicek[2] from Radiumhemmet in Sweden. There were no significant complications. Although hematomas formed, they did not produce discomfort and there was no mention of the necessity for evacuation or occurrence of secondary infection. They emphasized that there was no clinical evidence for seeding of tumor along the needle tract, and that this was not expected because of subsequent wide surgical excision or irradiation. They additionally referred to the classical work of Berg and Robbins at Memorial Hospital. Survival times were analyzed for 1406 patients subjected to radical surgery; 370 patients with breast carcinoma diagnosed by fine needle aspiration biopsy were compared to an equal control group and no statistical differences in morbidity or mortality were determined for a 10-year period, indicating, as Kline and Neal emphasized, that "the fear of dissemination of tumor cells through the needle tract with a worsening in prognosis is statistically unfounded." Bibbo and Zuspan[4] found no complications in 120 breast aspirates. In Frable's[5] personal experience with 469 cases, 127 breast tumors were aspirated without complication.

The development of precise criteria with unversality of data points for a cytological diagnosis of malignancy has helped to minimize the false positive diagnosis and report. In Franzen and Zajicek's mammoth resumé, only one false positive case was reported and review of the material confirmed the presence of malignant cells on the aspirate smears with incomplete sampling of the mastectomy specimen, which was discarded before further analysis could be done. There were no false positives in Hajdu and Melamed's[6] report of 315 cases from Memorial Hospital diagnosed as malignant by aspiration and confirmed histologically. Kern and Dermer[7] reviewed the cytological specimens from 535 patients and found no false positives among the aspiration biopsies. Similar experience from the University of Chicago[4] reinforced security in the technique. Frable reported two cases as false positives, but these had appropriately been signed out as "suspicious for carcinoma" and therapy had not been instituted. The retrospective reasons for these reports were diagnoses based on insufficient material and misinterpretation of the severe atypia that accompanies inflammation and repair. This experience has contributed useful caveats to the cytopathologist

TABLE I
FRANZÉN and ZAJICEK
Cytologic Findings in 1713 Breasts with Subsequent Histologic Diagnoses

Cytologic Findings	Histologic diagnoses			
	Benign lesion (807 cases)	"Precancerous lesion" including intraductal carcinoma (33 cases)	Carcinoma (873 cases)	Total (1713 cases)
	%	%	%	
Fat, blood or no yield	11.9	3.0	3.3	126
Cystic fluid	26.6	21.2	0.7	228
Inflammatory cells	4.2			34
Benign epithelium	32.5	39.4	4.5	314
Fibroadenoma	17.5	9.1	0.3	147
Cellular atypia	4.3	3.0	1.9	53
Carcinoma suspected	2.9	12.1	13.4	144
Carcinoma	0.1	12.1	75.8	667

[a]From *Acta Radiol.* **7**(4):241–262, 1968. Reproduced with permission.

interpreting needle aspirates. That therapy had not been predicated on these reports is an illustration that close rapport between the cytopathologist and clinician results in optimal patient care.

Frable expressed concern that the needle aspiration biopsy has been criticized because of its false negative rate, but emphasized the acceptability of the false negative statistic in a number of comprehensive series and reiterated that "a negative aspiration indicates only that a repeat aspiration may be necessary or that some other biopsy procedure is required." This applies, of course, to the clinical situation in which there is a high index of suspicion for malignant disease. In his series of breast aspirates, the false negative rate was 7%, which he considered representative of the average. Table I illustrates the statistical summary from the Radiumhemmet with an approximate false negative rate of 10%.

Kreuzer and Zajicek[8] were conscious of the problem of the false negative diagnosis and referred to the figures of 7.4–23.8% in the literature. They explored the factors responsible for the false negative diagnosis by reanalyzing 300 smears in groups of 100 from histologically proved cancers. The smears were segregated according to the initial interpretations of benign, suspicious, and conclusive for malignancy. The reasons for the inappropriate diagnoses were summarized. There was no relationship to clinical impression, contrary to the report by Rimsten et al.[1] "Clinical findings did not influence formulation of the cytologic report." Failure to report carcinoma cells was in part the product of suboptimal cellular sample and partially a reflection of lack of confident cellular identifica-

tion. The cell sample was compromised if the lesion was a small target (less than 1 cm in diameter), if the lesion was positioned adjacent to a cyst that was penetrated by the needle and intercepted harvest of the malignant sample, and if the tumor was either hypocellular or cellular detachment was restricted by desmoplastic fibrosis.

The false negative rate can be minimized by experience, and according to Franzen and Zajicek, if the pathologist who interprets the smears also performs the biopsy. They evaluated their improvement in accuracy as an expression of cumulative experience by comparing their results in 1962 (false negative rate of 7.9%) with their total result (1955–1963) of 10.8%. This, of course, corresponds to Frable's rate and an acceptable level.

A total of 276 breast aspirates were performed during a 3-year period (1978 through 1980) at the Eisenhower Medical Center, coordinated with 77 biopsies or mastectomies. The results are summarized in Table II, which illustrates the relationship between the projected diagnosis from the cytological impression and the subsequent tissue diagnosis. Malignant cells were identified in 37 aspirates and surgical follow-up was achieved in 33 cases by mastectomy and 2 cases by excisional biopsy. Confirmatory frozen section was obtained prior to mastectomy in 12 of the 33 cases. A malignant diagnosis was confirmed in 34 of 35 cases. The one discordant situation was a small incisional biopsy in which fibrocystic disease and inflammatory atypia were observed with ambiguity perpetuated by unavailability of the entire breast or a more substantial biopsy for evaluation. In two-thirds

TABLE II

Comparison of Cytological and Histological Diagnoses in 276 Breast Aspirates at the Eisenhower Medical Center, 1978–1980

Cytological diagnosis	Total number of cases	Number with surgical follow-up	Histological diagnoses		
			Benign	Atypical	Carcinoma
Unsatisfactory	70	12	8	0	4
Negative for malignancy	141	11	8	0	3
Atypical cells present	28	19	5	4	10
Malignant cells identified	37	35	1	0	34
			(bx only)		
Total	276	77	22	4	51

TABLE III
Histological Types of the Proved Carcinomas

Infiltrating duct cell	39
Medullary	3
Colloid	4
Adenosquamous	1
Tubular	1
Infiltrating lobular	3
Total	51

of the mastectomies definitive surgery was based exclusively on the needle aspirate report. In the 12 cases in which frozen section confirmation preceded mastectomy, the frozen section was performed either at the request of the pathologist or because the surgeon was familiarizing himself with the aspirate technic and had not yet developed full confidence in its predictive value. Of 141 aspirates interpreted as negative for malignancy, only 11 cases were submitted for surgical follow-up, despite the caveat that a negative aspirate does not exclude malignancy, particularly if there is a high clinical index of suspicion for cancer. Three carcinomas were unmasked. The numbers are too restricted for calculation of a statistically significant false negative rate, but the cytological slides were reviewed to establish the reasons for the inadequate diagnoses. In one case, too few cells were present for a reliable diagnosis and the smears should have been classified as "unsatisfactory" on this basis. The other two aspirates demonstrated adequate numbers of benign epithelial cells, implicating a sampling error, that is, failure of the needle to penetrate the cancer and retrieve representative cells. In 28 cases in which the cytological appearance was suspicious, but inconclusive for a malignant diagnosis, the tissue coordinates demonstrated unequivocal cancer in 10 cases and atypical intraductal hyperplasia in four. Four cancers detected as a consequence of excisional biopsy among 12 of the 70 unsatisfactory aspirates subjected to surgical intervention were overlooked because poor sampling failed to provide adequate material for cytological study.

Table III summarizes the histoarchitectural patterns of the proved carcinomas, examples of which follow in this chapter.

Clinical experience in the interpretation of the breast aspirate was initiated through examination of tissue specimens at the surgical bench with coordination of a reference library of slides to encourage comparisons between the cytological appearance and the more familiar histoarchitectual features. The simple mastectomy specimen that rescinded an exophytic fungating mass (Fig. 3-4) and provided cosmetic relief donated its renegade cells to the inquisitive needle probe.

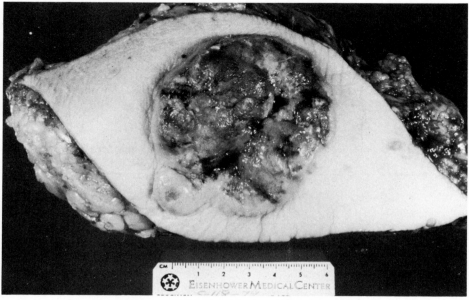

Fig. 3-4. Simple mastectomy specimen for debulking of an exophytic fungating ulcerated mass.

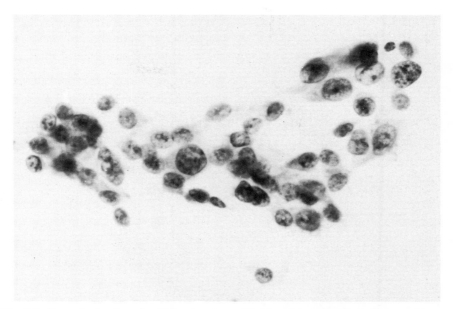

Fig. 3-5. Papanicolaou's stain, 625×, cytology of infiltrating duct cell carcinoma of breast.

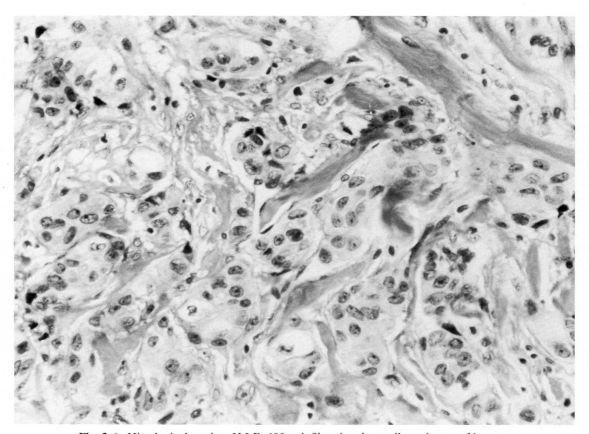

Fig. 3-6. Histological section, H&E, 400×, infiltrating duct cell carcinoma of breast.

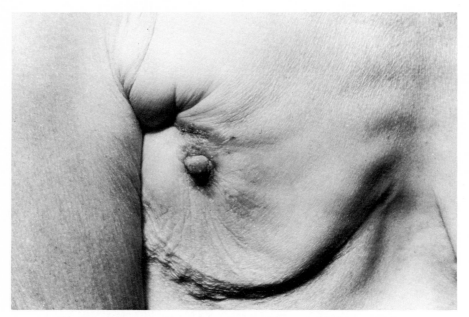

Fig. 3-7. Clinically advanced carcinoma of breast with skin retraction.

Cell clusters were abundant, but loosely cohesive (Fig. 3-5) and nuclear features were incongruously bland with respect to the variegated pleomorphism of the aggressive gross lesion. Chromatin appeared finely stippled and gently dispersed with erratic organization into chromo- centers. Nuclear boundaries appeared distinct and smooth without noticeable serrations or molding of adjacent membranes. Variations in size and more subtle discrepancies in shape could be detected and despite ulceration at the surface of the lesion the smear was spared a background

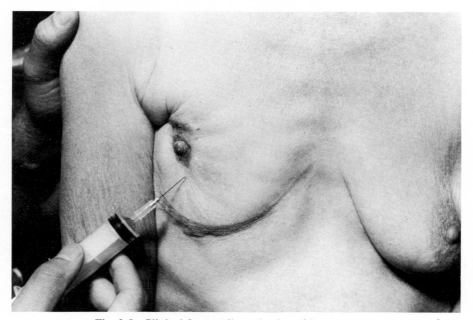

Fig. 3-8. Clinical fine needle aspiration of breast tumor.

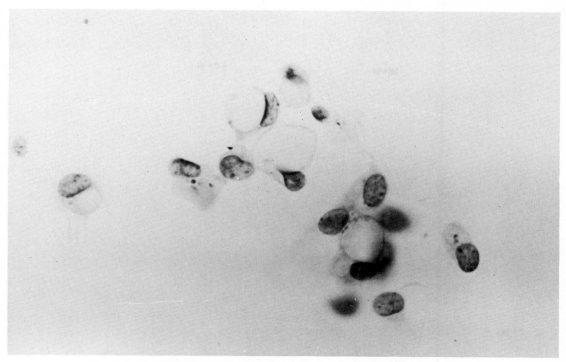

Fig. 3-9. Needle aspirate, Papanicolaou's stain, 625×, signet ring carcinoma.

diathesis and inflammatory exudate. The tissue sections further emphasized the rather uniform bland nuclei of polyhedral cells herded by coarse collagen bands into arbitrary mosaic nests (Fig. 3-6).

The inaugural patient referred for breast aspiration was a 61-year-old female who cohabitated with her tumor for 10 years until progressive dyspnea and unrelenting spinal pain influenced her to consult a physician. The clinican insisted on a tissue diagnosis prior to initiation of chemotherapy, despite the obvious induration, stellate retraction, and axillary excursion of the breast with an incompressibly indurated subareolar mass (Fig. 3-7). The patient refused incisional biopsy, but acquiesced to aspiration, which was performed by the pathologist in his office without preliminary local anesthesia (Fig. 3-8). The cells contained mucicarmine-positive cytoplasmic vacuoles, which displaced the vesicular, rather bland nuclei peripherally, creating the configuration of dissociated signet rings (Fig. 3-9). It was initially considered that the signet ring pattern was consistent with slow growth and long duration of the tumor and that, despite the bland nuclear characteristics, the aspirate was diagnostic for malignancy. Combined systemic chemotherapy was initiated, but the patient died with cavitary pneumonitis and disseminated tumor. At necropsy examination, the carcinoma was confirmed as an indurated mass with serrated margins, measuring 4 by 3 by 2 cm with infiltration of muscle and skin (Fig. 3-10) and extensive metastatic involvement of spine (Fig. 3-11a) correlative with the presenting complaint of back pain. The histological sections demonstrated a poorly differentiated infiltrating duct cell carcinoma in which the signet ring configuration was a minimal component. (Fig. 3–11b) Sheets, anastomosing cords, trabeculae, and abortive acini were dominant. This noncorrelative finding aroused awareness that the cellular sample may correctly substantiate a malignancy without conforming exclusively to the histological structure, particularly when derived from a mixed pattern. This problem of sampling vindicates repeated passes to assess variable areas of the tumor.

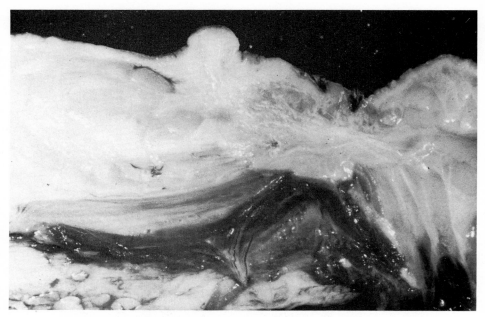

Fig. 3-10. Gross specimen, sagittal section of breast carcinoma at autopsy.

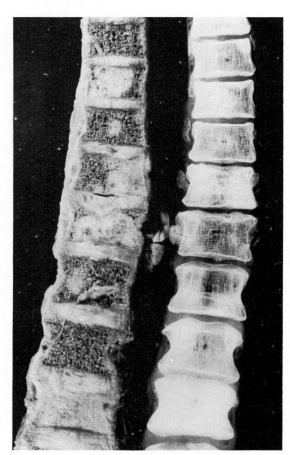

Fig. 3-11 a. Gross specimen and specimen radiograph demonstrating metastatic breast carcinoma in spine.

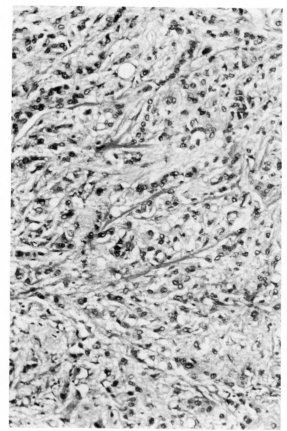

Fig. 3-11 b. Histological section, H&E, 160×, histology of the primary breast carcinoma.

PRIMARY DIAGNOSIS: COMMON AND EXTRAORDINARY LESIONS

Infiltrating duct cell carcinoma is the most frequently aspirated malignancy of the breast in our community hospital experience. The cytomorphological characteristics are consistent despite variations in nuclear grade, so that an accurate assessment for the reliable prediction of cancer is possible from an adequate preparation. Figure 3-12 illustrated the mammographic appearance of a palpable and clinically suspicious mass in the lower-outer quadrant of the right breast in a 64-year-old woman. A fine needle aspirate (Fig. 3-13) demonstrated malignant cells and modified radical mastectomy was elected. The mastectomy specimen (Fig. 3-14) demonstrates the proximity of the lesion to the skin and its accessibility to the needle. The

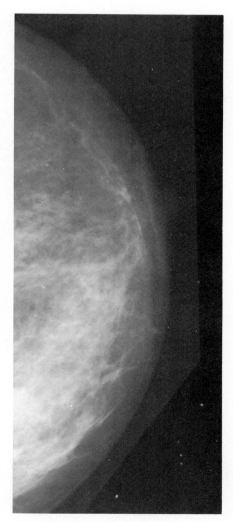

Fig. 3-12. Clinical mammogram demonstrating the 1-cm mass in proximity to the surface.

tumor appeared well delineated, but unencapsulated, 1.2 cm. in diameter, with a homogeneous solid substance and a gentle scalloped periphery. The cellular features amplified by Papanicolaou's stain are characteristic of duct cell carcinoma and correspond to conventional criteria.[7,9,10] The stereoscopic perspective of the smear demonstrates abundant cellularity with a tendency to aggregation that is distracted by the preponderant isolation of dissociated cells. Although fortuitous formations occur, linear associates are more reminiscent of how the cells related in trabecular cords among collagenous fibers in tissue confluence (Fig. 3-15). Pleomor-

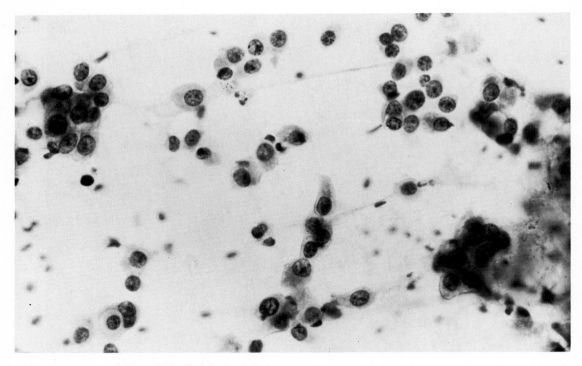

Fig. 3-13. Needle aspirate, Papanicolaou's stain, 500×, cytology of infiltrating duct cell carcinoma.

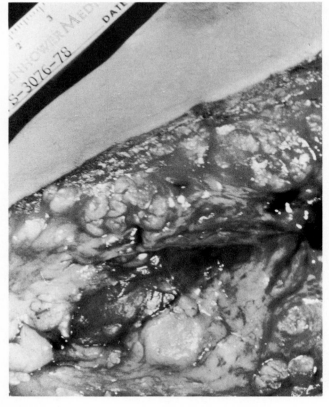

Fig. 3-14. Mastectomy specimen incorporating the small carcinoma corresponding to the clinical mammogram.

phism is subtle, reflecting variations in nuclear size and shape. Cytoplasm is variable in amount, granular or homogenized, and delineated by crisp margins. This photographic document, recapitulating others in this chapter, contradicts Schondorf's proclamation[10] that the process of aspiration destroys cytoplasm that is absent from most malignant cells in breast aspirates. The cytoplasmic component accentuated by Papanicolaou's stain permits analysis of relationships among cells (nuclear molding, acinar and trabecular formations) and provides insight into certain details of function, such as mucus production with elaboration into vacuolar envelopes. Chromatin is coarse, often condensed and erratically distributed, leaving residues of vacuous nucleoplasm to highlight nucleoli. Nucleoli may be variable in number, size, and morphology with spiculation and angularity. Serrational convolutional folding of nuclear envelopes is not present in this case, but can be observed in breast aspirates from high-grade malignancies.

The similarity of this cellular population to the aspirated cells (Fig. 3-16) from a 1.0 cm. breast carcinoma resected from a 55-year-old female emphasizes the universality of these criteria. The gross characteristics of the tumor were dissimilar (Fig. 3-17): the peripheral margin appears stellately infiltrative and an intricate labyrinthine pattern of necrosis punctuates the transected surface. The histological sections supplement the aspirate in dramatizing the nuclear architecture (Fig. 3-18), providing images of recalcitrant nucleoli and resurgent chromatin particles. Figure 3-19 is a final example of the mastectomy for duct cell carcinoma, corresponding to singly disported cells with anisokaryosis, hyperchromasia, coarse chromatin dispersion, and nucleolar prominence collected by aspiration biopsy (Fig. 3-20) and confirmed histologically (Fig. 3-21).

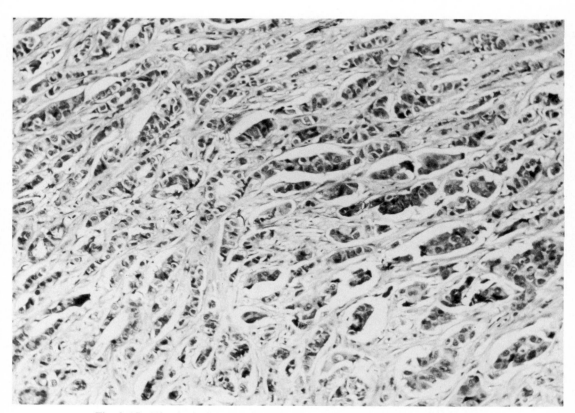

Fig. 3-15. Histological section, H&E, 160×, infiltrating duct cell carcinoma.

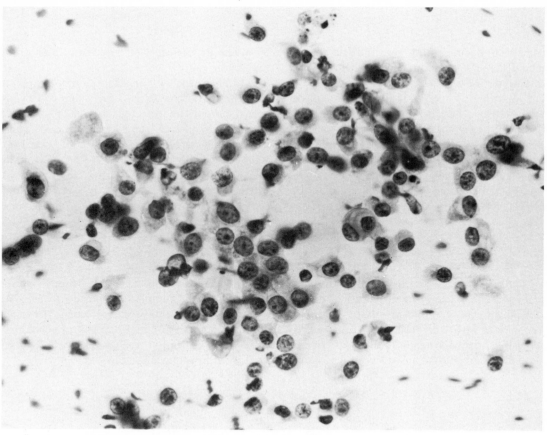

Fig. 3-16. Needle aspirate, Papanicolaou's stain, 500×, infiltrating duct cell carcinoma.

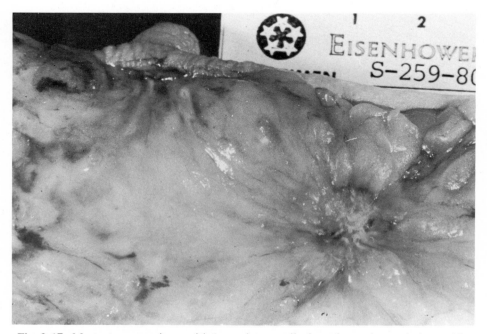

Fig. 3-17. Mastectomy specimen with 1-cm circumscribed carcinoma in proximity to skin.

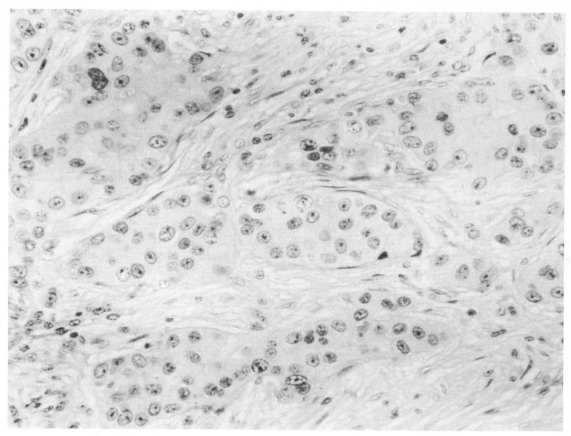

Fig. 3-18. Histological section, H&E, 160×, infiltrating duct cell carcinoma.

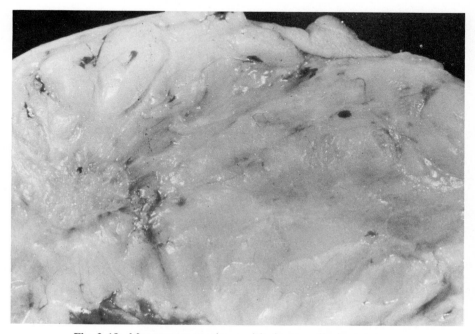

Fig. 3-19. Mastectomy specimen with circumscribed carcinoma.

The diagnostic criteria for breast carcinoma by fine needle aspiration are defined empirically for duct cell carcinoma because of its frequency and the absence of peculiarities of format. Schondorf[10] relies heavily on nuclear enlargement and pleomorphism but accepts the loss of cellular cohesiveness as a differential clue, assigning this feature and increased cellularity to "indirect" properties of malignancy. Kern and Dermer[7] emphasize nuclear enlargement, hyperchromasia, pleomorphism, prominent nucleoli, irregular chromatin, and sheeted aggregation with peripheral dyscohesion as reliable indices. Mouriquand and Pasquier[9] concur with these criteria, which they have creatively applied to a cytological grading method for fine needle aspiration smears. Smears from 178 histologically confirmed breast cancers were assigned to one of three categories of nuclear differentiation (I, well-differentiated, through III, anaplastic) and then correlated with the clinical course for a 1 year follow-up. In grade I carcinomas, the cells were observed in clusters and exhibited rather bland nuclear features and uniformity that discouraged a malignant diagnosis; Grade II carcinomas presented isolated cells satellite to cohesive clusters with irregular chromatin and enlarged nuclei; Grade III cells were predominantly isolated units with minimal community, overt nuclear features of malignancy, and frequent naked nuclei. Sixty-six percent of the Grade III tumors experienced an unfavorable outcome, compared with 8.9% of Grade II and only 4% of Grade I lesions. Their conclusions incorporate as the factors of prognostic significance decreased cellular cohesion, increased nuclear and nucleolar size, frequent nucleolar number, protrusions of the nuclear envelope, hypochromasia and perhaps intracytoplasmic "bull's-eye" vacuoles. Cytoprognostic factors are extensions of diagnostic criteria dynamically applied to tumor behavior.

Our developing experience with fine needle aspiration cytology has embraced characteristic examples of variants of infiltrating duct cell carcinoma, dignified by separate terminology because of peculiar characteristics or morphology, macroarchitecture, cellular product, or clinical behavior. We have had the opportunity, although limited, to examine colloid, medullary,

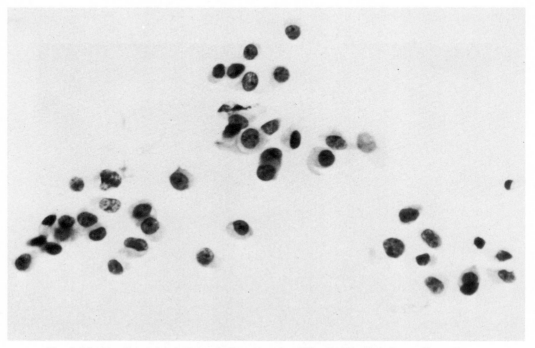

Fig. 3-20. Needle aspirate, Papanicolaou's stain, 625×, infiltrating duct cell carcinoma.

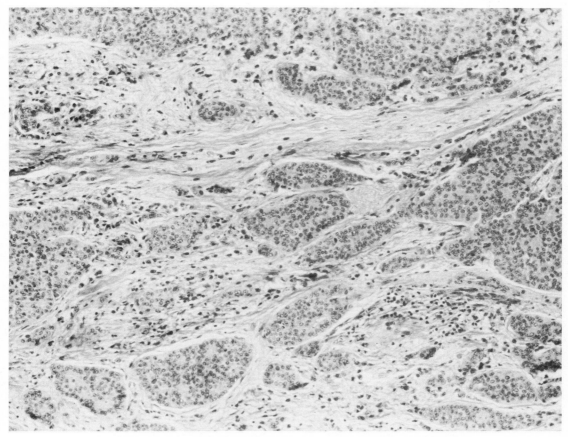

Fig. 3-21. Histological section, H&E, 160×, infiltrating duct cell carcinoma.

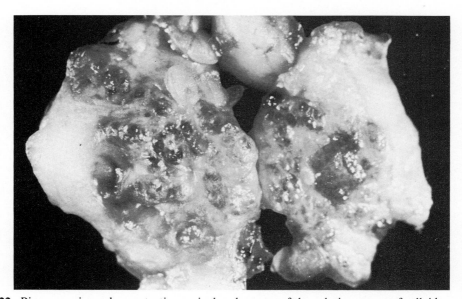

Fig. 3-22. Biopsy specimen demonstrating vesicular character of the gelatinous type of colloid carcinoma.

tubular, adenosquamous, and metaplastic carcinomas by this method, in addition to one male breast carcinoma of ductal origin. The examples that follow are the representative products of specimen or clinical aspirates collected during a 3-year period of active clinical application.

Colloid or mucinous carcinoma is a distinct histological entity, which may develop as a pure lesion or as a component of a mixed pattern. Pure mucinous lesions occur in older women, have a long gestation, exhibit a "pushing" rather than a stellately infiltrative margin, are associated with less frequent axillary metastases and appreciably increased survival.[11] Figure 3-22 demonstrates a 3.0 cm gelatinous, vesicular mass from the right breast of a 54-year-old woman. The lobulated character of the mucoid parenchyma is apparent and the margin is gently undulating. Variation may be imparted by interspersed hemorrhagic extravasation and reticular fibrosis, but overt necrosis is not observed. The needle aspirate (Fig. 3-23) incorporates as a suspension matrix for the cells a pale, homogeneous, often dusky, blue-gray fibrillar extracellular material that may be confirmed as mucus by appropriate histochemical stains. The cells are distributed in insular aggregates and detached isolates, but where community organization is observed, there is affinity for contact and even molding. Nuclear shape is rather uniform, chromatin punctate, and stippled, and nucleoli prominent and single. Other areas of the lesion may demonstrate vagarious nuclei that are more hyperchromatic, angular, and less adamant in their preference for cellular coalition (Fig. 3-24). The mucoid milieu with its suspended cellular composites is best appreciated in the histological sections (Fig. 3-25), where relationship between stroma, external mucus, and cellular components can be examined. Note that the mucus is extravasated and that cytoplasmic vacuoles are not a feature.

Medullary carcinoma should be recognized as a clinicopathological entity because of its distinctively favorable prognosis evidenced by a projected 10-year survival of 84%, despite the

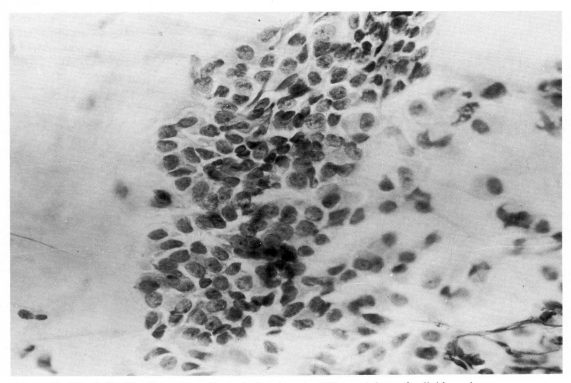

Fig. 3-23. Needle aspirate, Papanicolaou's stain, 500×, cytology of colloid carcinoma.

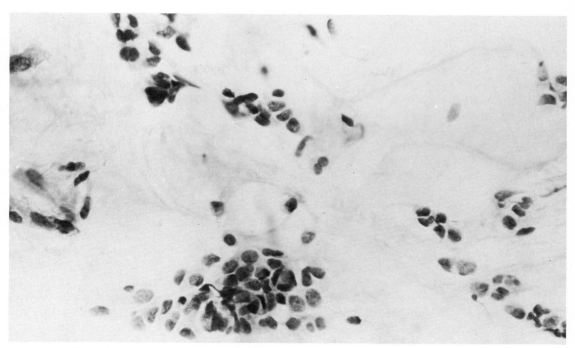

Fig. 3-24. Needle aspirate, Papanicolaou's stain, 500×, cytology of colloid carcinoma.

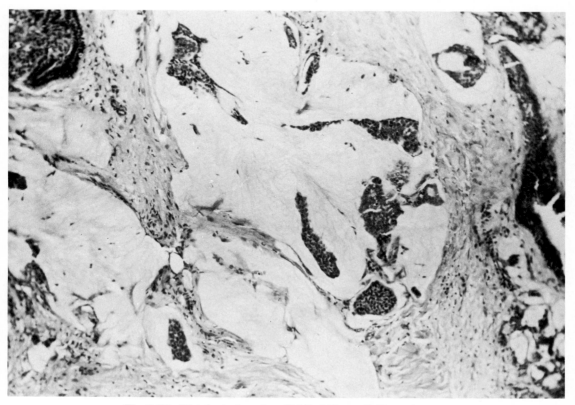

Fig. 3-25. Histological section, H&E, 160×, colloid carcinoma.

presence of axillary node metastases.[12] Stringent diagnostic criteria must prevail if the lesion is to be classified appropriately for prophetic value. Azzopardi[12] refers to the criteria of Ridolfi et al.[13] for medullary carcinoma: the tumor must be sharply and completely circumscribed grossly and microscopically, a syncytial growth pattern must constitute at least 75% of the lesion sampled, a mononuclear stromal infiltrate must be substantial and diffuse, and the malignant cells should be larger than most breast carcinoma cells with unequivocal nuclear features of cancer. The aspirates featured in Figures 3-26 and 3-27 are from a 38-year-old female with a nontender mass in the right breast. Palpatory characteristics of circumscription and mobility had clinically suggested fibroadenoma, but the cellular population contradicted this postulate. There is an intimately comingled biphasic population of cells in which the epithelial component is dominant and portrays a syncytial quality projected by the juxtaposition of cells with indef-

inite cytoplasmic boundaries. The abundant cytoplasm is pale, vesicular, and delicately granular. Nuclear characteristics vary from vesicular with bland, finely stippled chromatin and inconspicuous nucleoli to hyperchromatic with coarsely precipitated chromatin substance, prominent nucleoli, and serrational convolutions of nuclear envelopes. Interspersed are lymphocytes distributed between cells as adamant cohabitants. The histological sections correspond with veracity (Fig. 3-28). The epithelial component is sheeted, exhibiting indistinct cytoplasm and pale, vesicular nuclei with atypia that conforms to malignant criteria. The lymphoid population is focally intensified by condensation into pseudofollicles at foci of trabecular interruption but can be seen in random distribution among epithelial constituents.

Another example (Fig. 3-29) reflects features of nuclear anaplasia in which anisokaryosis, nucleolar multiplicity, and hyperchromasia may occur despite the presence of other features

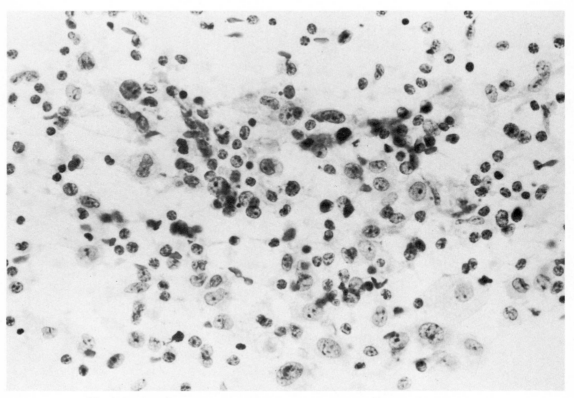

Fig. 3-26. Needle aspirate, Papanicolaou's stain, 500×, medullary carcinoma.

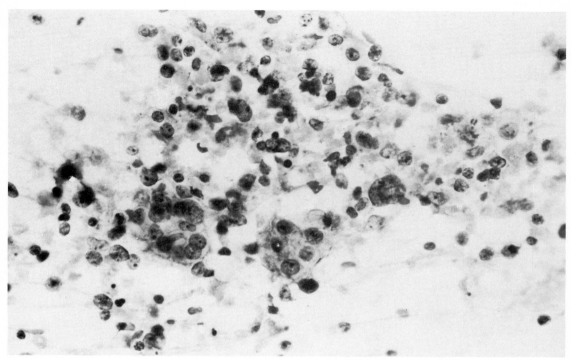

Fig. 3-27. Needle aspirate, Papanicolaou's stain, reduced from 500×, medullary carcinoma.

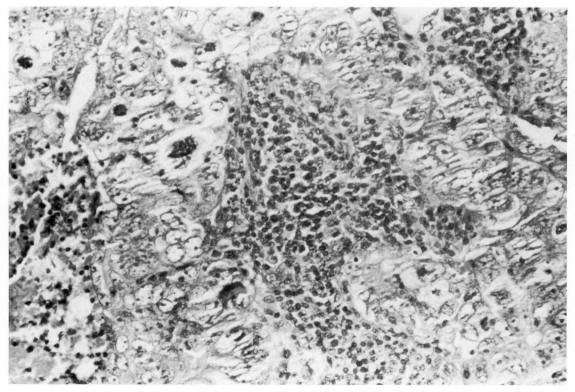

Fig. 3-28. Histological section, H&E, 400×, medullary carcinoma.

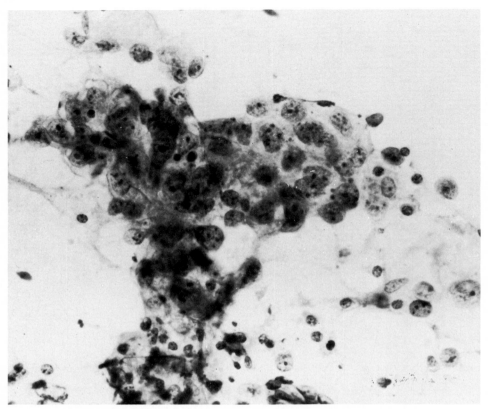

Fig. 3-29. Needle aspirate, Papanicolaou's stain, 500×, medullary carcinoma.

consistent with medullary differentiation. The histological pattern (Fig. 3-30) corresponds and conforms to Fisher et al.'s[11] summary of the characteristics of this breast cancer variant: the nuclear grade is usually I, the histological grade often III; mucin is absent; elastic deposition in the stroma is negligible; lymphatic invasion is usually absent; there is no intraductal component; necrosis is marked; the patients are usually between the ages of 20 and 44 years. The lymphoid population is assumed to mediate an immune response that confers the improved prognosis.

Infiltrating duct cell carcinoma of the breast may be associated with cartilaginous or osseous differentiation as an extraordinary and infrequent phenomenon. The rarity of the lesion explains the paucity of information concerning its cytological characteristics in the medium of the needle aspirate preparation. We have had the fortuitous opportunity to examine one case by this method from the surgical specimen. A 32-year-old postpartum woman consulted a surgeon for evaluation of a 3.0 cm mass in the upper quadrant of the right breast. He excised the lesion under local anesthesia and submitted the tissue for confirmation of what he judged to represent an organizing breast abscess. The histological confirmation of infiltrating duct cell carcinoma with cartilaginous "metaplasia" resulted in a modified radical mastectomy without excision of the internal mammary chain, and it was the mastectomy specimen that donated cells for study. The residual tumor (Fig. 3-31) appeared irregularly nodular, resilient, gritty, with lobulations and punctate foci of yellow softening. The biphasic population of cells exhibits subtle variations in character, but sufficient divergence is present to permit a distinction (Fig. 3-32). A nodular aggregate of small cells with hyperchromatic nuclei and condensed cytoplasm (arrow) exhibits irregularities of nuclear membranes and molding with sharp, angular protrusions. These are considered the aberrant ductal

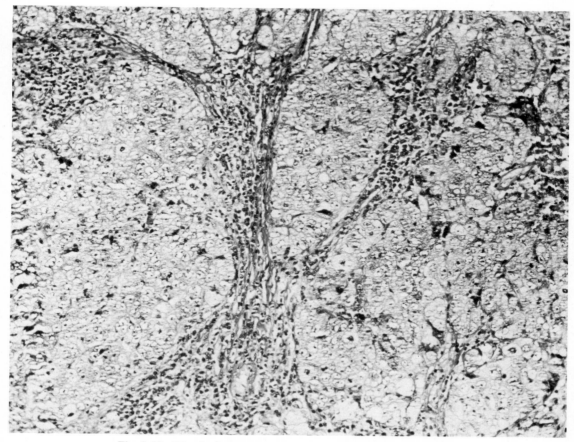

Fig. 3-30. Histological section, H & E, 160×, medullary carcinoma.

epithelial cells, which are couched by a crescent of larger cells with pale, abundant, vesicular cytoplasm and nuclei that appear less condensed, enhancing the coarsely stippled chromatinic pattern. These are interpreted as the cartilaginous element. These features are further amplified: Figure 3-33 demonstrates the epithelial component in which cytoplasmic membranes are sharply delineated, and the mosaic arrangement descries the absence of syncytial distribution. The nuclei are uniform in their aberration from normalcy, exhibiting elusive, jagged sculptures in their membranes, prominent nucleoli and irregular dispersement of chromatinic substance. This corresponds with identity to the mosaic sheets of malignant ductal cells in the histological section (Fig. 3-34). The second population is distinguished by its syncytial confluence, the larger nuclei and the coarse chromatin pattern

with parachromatin clearing and blatant aniso-karyosis (Figure 3-35). This cluster corresponds to the cartilaginous differentiation of the tissue where the stromal matrix confers the image of cell dispersion in a syncytial milieu that interrupts the homogeneity of the tumor structure almost cataclysmically.

Smith and Taylor[14] have advanced the controversial postulate that cartilaginous metaplasia occurs from both the ductal epithelial elements and from the stroma. When the epithelial element is an infiltrating duct cell carcinoma, it is the epithelium that contributes the metaplastic element, and the cartilage may assume a malignant or benign pattern. Intraductal papillomas and cystosarcoma phyllodes associated with metaplastic conversion produce the cartilaginous element from the stroma. In this case, there is some resemblance of the "metaplastic"

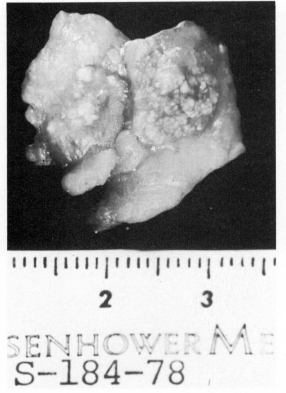

Fig. 3-31. Gross specimen, duct cell carcinoma with cartilaginous "metaplasia."

cells to the carcinoma and the cartilaginous constituent is cytologically cancerous. The presence of bone or cartilage is not expected to alter the behavior of the lesion when compared to lesions in which they are not a component. The patient has survived 3 years without recurrence or metastasis.

Duct cell carcinoma of the breast in its metaplastic posture can assume characteristics in mimicry of squamous carcinoma, the prognostic significance of which is undetermined. Azzopardi[12] has concluded that pure squamous cell carcinoma of the breast is exceedingly rare and that most lesions assigned to this diagnostic category are adenocarcinomas exhibiting variable effort at squamous metaplasia. When clearly defined glandular patterns are juxtaposed to foci of malignant squamous change, the possibility of coincidental differential lineages is implicated. Adenosquamous carcinoma as a diagnostic term may provoke semantic conflicts, because there is the implicit concern that cytogenesis be accurately represented by the terminology that describes its cellular products.

We have chosen to interpret our examples of squamous differentiation in association with adenocarcinoma of the breast as adenosquamous carcinoma, in full cognizance that the subscribers to the metaplastic philosophy may be equally

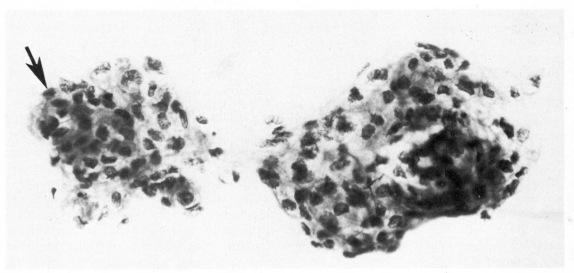

Fig. 3-32. Needle aspirate, Papanicolaou's stain, 312.5×, duct cell carcinoma with cartilaginous "metaplasia."

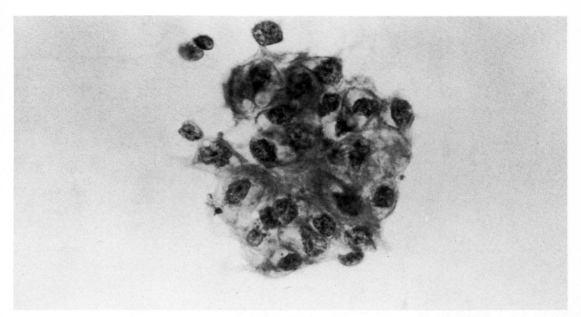

Fig. 3-33. Needle aspirate, Papanicolaou's stain, 500×, duct cell carcinoma with cartilaginous "metaplasia."

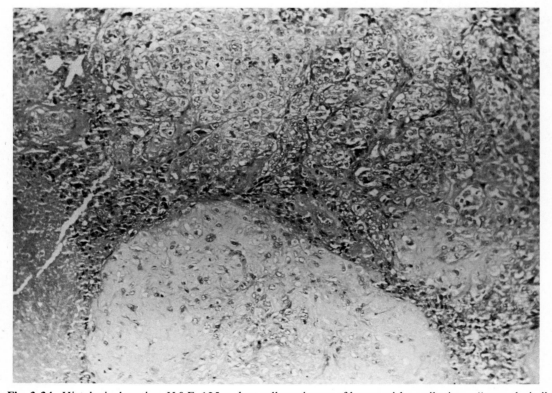

Fig. 3-34. Histological section, H&E, 125×, duct cell carcinoma of breast with cartilaginous "metaplasia."

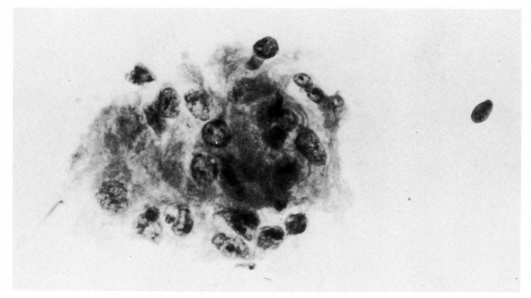

Fig. 3-35. Needle aspirate, Papanicolaou's stain, 500×, "metaplastic" component.

justified. A fine needle aspirate was performed to evaluate a 5.0 cm mass in the tail of Spence in the left breast of a 72-year-old woman who had sustained a right radical mastectomy at age 68 for infiltrating small cell undifferentiated carcinoma. A bimorphic cellular population was retrieved (Fig. 3-36). Cohesive clusters resemble abortive acinar structures with pale, slightly granular cytoplasm surrounding vesicular nuclei with prominent nucleoli and perinucleolar halos. These are considered the glandular derivatives of the tumor. Adjacent cells provide a separatist element of different qualities. The nuclei appear densely hyperchromatic and angular with ho-

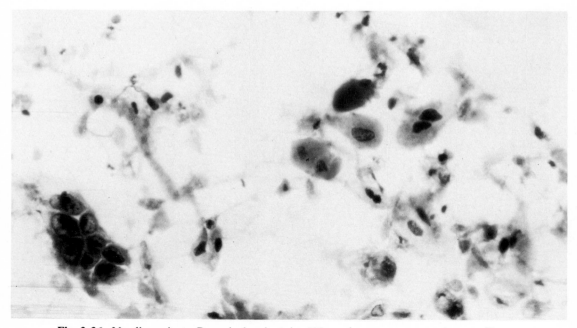

Fig. 3-36. Needle aspirate, Papanicolaou's stain, 400×, adenosquamous carcinoma of breast.

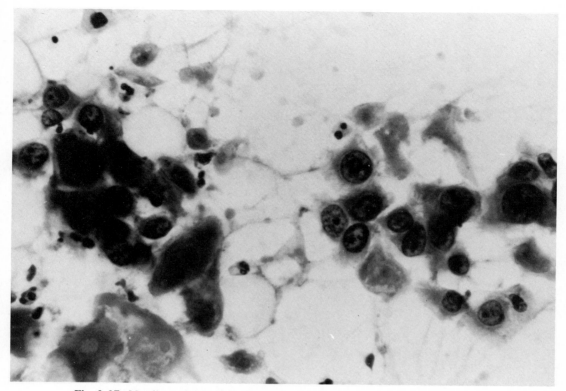

Fig. 3-37. Needle aspirate, Papanicolaou's stain, 625×, adenosquamous carcinoma.

mogenization of the chromatin particles. Cytoplasm is dense, eosinophilic, hyalinized, as if impregnated with keratinaceous protein. When these cells relate in aggregates, a pavemented mosaic is created, acknowledging the squamous component of the neoplasm (Fig. 3-37). The modified radical mastectomy specimen incorporated a 5 by 3 by 2 cm incompressibly indurated neoplasm with smooth, scalloped peripheral margins and central cavitary necrosis. Microscopically the cells are arranged in abortive acini and pavemented sheets recapitulating glandular and squamoid patterns (Fig. 3-38). Mucicarmine-positive cellular products were confirmed within the acinar areas. The tumor was estrogen receptor-negative, but it is unknown whether the squamous change is related or responsible.

The male breast is susceptible to the epithelial malignancies that affect the female breast, including rare examples of infiltrating lobular carcinoma[15] despite the usual absence of terminal ducts and lobules in male mammary structure. Crichlow[16] reported that 2217 male breast carcinomas are documented in the literature of the 20th century and that this rare tumor constitutes only 1% of all carcinomas of the breast. Invariably there is a poor prognosis related to proximity to dermal lymphatics and the internal mammary chain, areolar involvement, late diagnosis with established metastases, and delayed therapy. The needle aspiration procedure can help to rectify this situation by providing earlier, rapid diagnosis if the male seeks immediate attention. The rules of cytointerpretation apply directly from composite knowledge of female breast cancer, but there may be more of a tendency for the malignant cells to aggregate. We examined a needle aspirate from a 5 cm subareolar, poorly defined mass in the left breast of a 56-year-old male. Nipple discharge, axillary adenopathy, and peau d'orange alternation of the skin were absent. The cells exhibit subtle changes of malignancy, including variability in shape, molding, and nucleolar prominence. Alignment in trabeculae two to three cell layers in width, or arrangements around a central lumi-

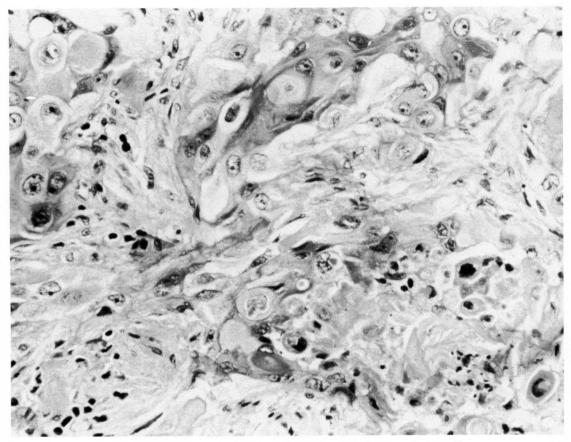

Fig. 3-38. Histological section, H&E, 400×, adenosquamous carcinoma of breast.

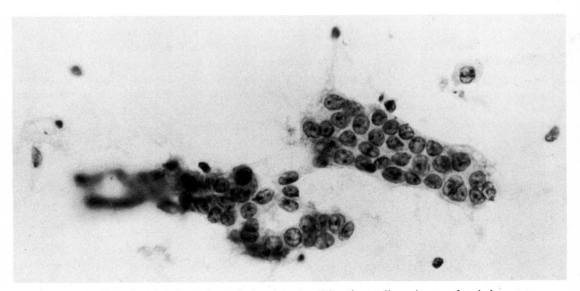

Fig. 3-39. Needle of aspirate, Papanicolaou's stain, 625×, duct cell carcinoma of male breast.

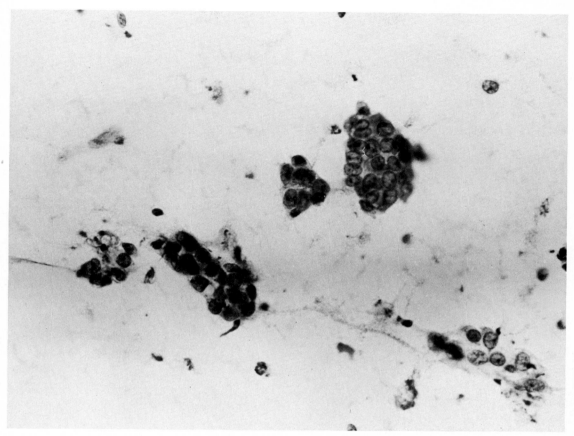

Fig. 3-40. Needle aspirate, Papanicolaou's stain, 500×, duct cell carcinoma of male breast.

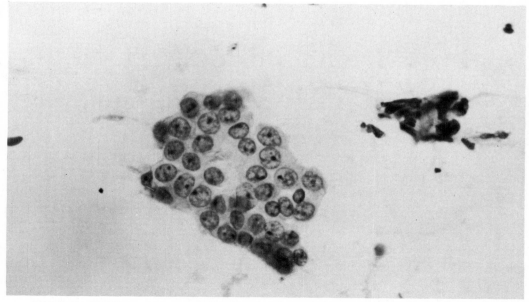

Fig. 3-41. Needle aspirate, Papanicolaou's stain, 500×, duct cell carcinoma of male breast.

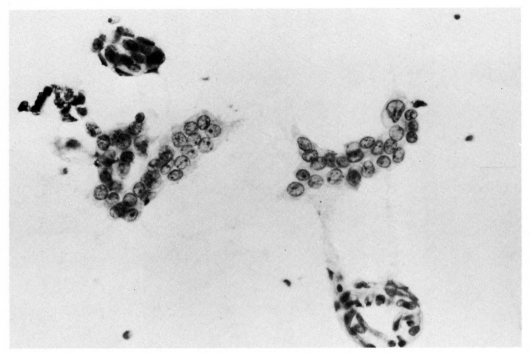

Fig. 3-42. Needle aspirate, Papanicolaou's stain, 625×, duct cell carcinoma of male breast.

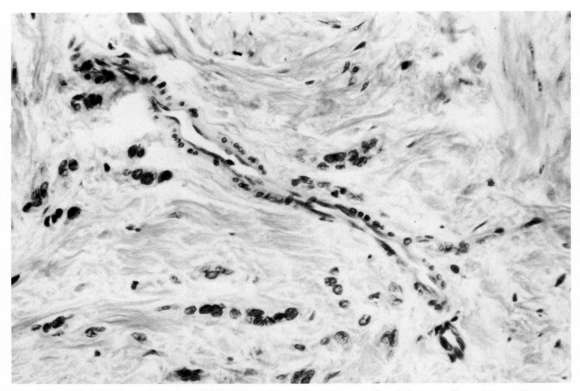

Fig. 3-43. Histological section, H&E, 400×, duct cell carcinoma of male breast adjacent to capillary.

nal space (Fig. 3-39, 3-40) are characteristic configurations indicative of preserved cohesiveness. One to three nucleoli are observed in the vesicular nucleoplasm. Nuclear membranes appear smooth, nonindented, and crisply defined (Fig. 3-41). Parallel linear aggregates of tumor cells juxtaposed to extracted capillaries with preserved endothelial cells can be observed for interesting comparisons (Fig. 3-42) and are exactly comparable to histological sections from the resection (Fig. 3-43). A radical mastectomy was the procedure used and the specimen contained a permeative, ill-defined tumor beneath the skin, restricted from pectoral involvement (Fig. 3-44) but accessible to the probing needle.

The reticence to diagnose tubular carcinoma in histological sections, particularly when the lesion is small, may be transferred to the aspirate investigation of the lesion, but satisfactory differential points exist to identify the entity and separate it from other forms of ductal cancer and from sclerosing adenosis. The cytological

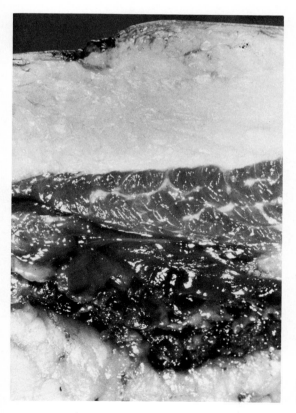

appearance of tubular carcinoma of the breast in needle aspiration was discussed by this author in the 1979 Diagnostic Seminar of the American Society of Cytology,[17] and Figure 3-45 is from that case.

The ductal cells of tubular carcinoma are uniform and bland, arranged as hollow, bifurcating casts of ductal templates. Nuclear detail is soporifically monotonous, vesicular, with punctate dispersion of chromatin. Histological sections may show occasional protrusion into luminal spaces as "apocrine snouts." The nuclear membranes are crisply outlined. Detached cells signify diminished cohesiveness, but the isolated cells maintain their ground-glass, uninteresting nuclear character. When adipose matrix is incorporated with epithelial aggregates, the relationship of epithelial cells to stroma is not intruded by myoepithelial elements. Therefore the presence of epithelium, although bland, in the midst of fat is an aggressive act. The lumina created by the proliferating cells are patulous and uniform in diameter. This is in contradistinction to the pseudoinfiltrative pattern of sclerosing adenosis in which luminal caliber is often irregular, reduced, or obliterated by glandular units distorted by circumscribing, retractile fibrosis. Tubular carcinoma has been recognized as a special variant of duct cell carcinoma because of its indolent behavior. Although it may be multifocal and bilateral, it rarely involves axillary lymph nodes. In 35 cases reported from the Memorial Hospital[18] there were no deaths related to the tumor. Carstens et al.[18] emphasized, however, that in 80% of their cases, other types of carcinoma coexisted in the same breast, predominantly intraductal papillary carcinoma. Prognosis was then considered to depend on the associated carcinoma, but this is somewhat enigmatic because 65% of the associated cancers were noninvasive intraductal papillary lesions. The concomitant development of tubular carcinoma and another type of breast cancer projects the possibility of incorporating a variegated cytological population in an aspiration biopsy, particularly if there are several

Fig. 3-44. Mastectomy specimen, male breast with obscure permeative tumor.

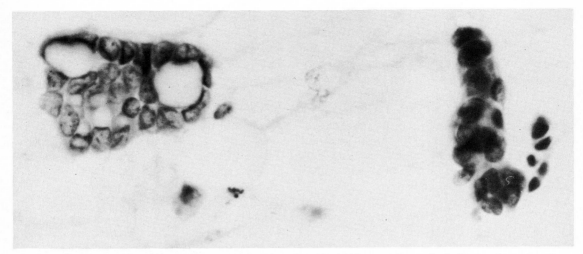

Fig. 3-45. Needle aspirate, Papanicolaou's stain, about 400×, cytology of tubular carcinoma.

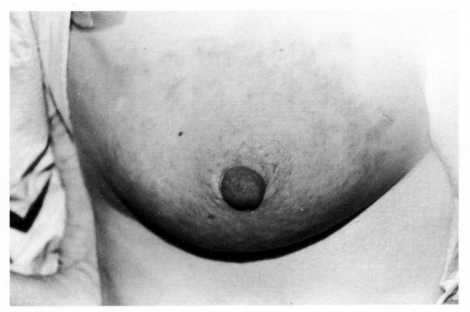

Fig. 3-46. Clinical photograph demonstrating inflammatory carcinoma of the breast.

passes from various regions of the tumor. The awareness of this factor should protect the cytopathologist from overlooking the tubular component if it is obscured by a more dominant lesion.

Aspiration biopsy is limited in evaluation of the patient with clinical inflammatory carcinoma of the breast because confirmation of this disease resides in the histopathological demonstration of dermal lymphatic carcinomatosis.[12] The disease is a special entity because of its fulminant course and the contraindication of surgical intervention. The clinical reaction is expressed by an erysipeloid granular hyperemia and hyperthermia of the skin of the breast (Fig. 3-46), which may be associated with a discrete mass in as many as two-thirds of the cases. The needle may be used to confirm the malignant character of the mass, but skin biopsy is essential to differentiate a cellulitis-type reaction from verified tumor emboli in lymphatics. In the case we feature, the patient is a 47-year-old female with the characteristic skin pattern and palpable homolateral axillary adenopathy. We used aspiration biopsy to examine the enlarged lymph nodes and cellular validation of metastatic carcinoma was obtained (Fig. 3-47). Hostile epithelial cells with enlarged, irregular nuclei, disturbed nuclear-cytoplasmic ratios, molding, and trabecular adhesion were extracted from the node. This information may help to guide therapy by contributing information of stage to the comprehensive perspective.

Invasive lobular carcinoma of the breast is a clinicopathological entity that deserves recognition and segregation from other types of breast cancer because of the unusually high incidence of bilaterality and the practical implications the diagnosis poses. This type may be associated with a lesser incidence of nodal metastases and short-term treatment failures, and its association with positive estrogen receptor proteins may influence treatment by hormonal manipulation.[12] The cytological diagnosis in needle aspirates resides in the bland uniformity of small cells situated in linear filaments reflecting their repose in concentric, targetoid enfilades in tissues. Figure 3-48 demonstrates four bland cells in such aggregation, magnified to illustrate the innocuous nucleoplasm with vague nucleoli and minimal cytoplasm. The tissue preparation reveals how these cells related in file among collagen bundles (Fig. 3-49), indicating the usual pattern of infiltrating lobular carcinoma. Alternative patterns have been described, particularly the confluent organization contributed by Fechner.[19]

Although the emphasis in this chapter has certainly been focused on the malignant breast lesion, brief reference to appearance of fibroadenoma and fibrocystic disease in the aspiration biopsy material is indicated.

Fibroadenoma is the most commonly aspirated benign tumor and generally presents as a discrete, resiliently indurated, mobile mass that is difficult to restrain under the penetrating needle (Fig. 3-50). The cellular derivatives are luxurient, tenaciously adherent in serpiginous and branching trabeculae that suggest casts of cleftular templates. Occasionally a dissociated cell will present a fusiform configuration, but the

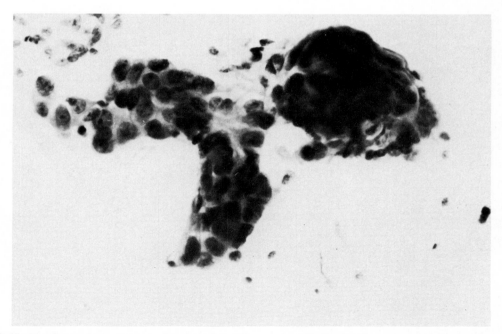

Fig. 3-47. Needle aspirate, Papanicolaou's stain, 400×, metastatic duct cell carcinoma of breast in axillary lymph node.

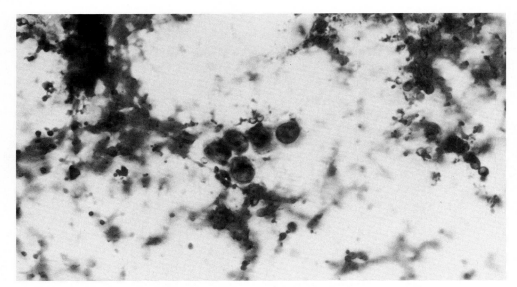

Fig. 3-48. Needle aspirate, Papanicolaou's stain 625×, cytology of invasive lobular carcinoma.

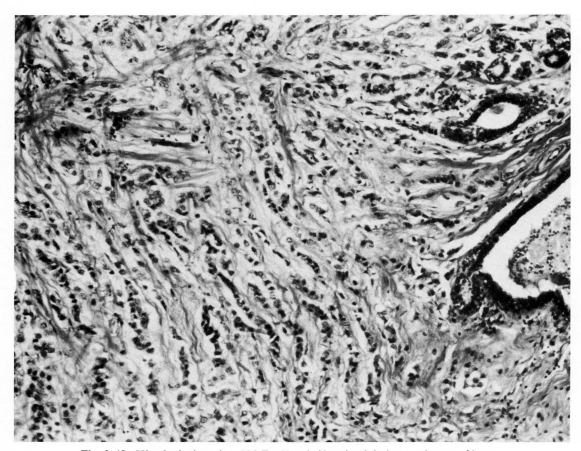

Fig. 3-49. Histological section, H&E 160×, infiltrating lobular carcinoma of breast.

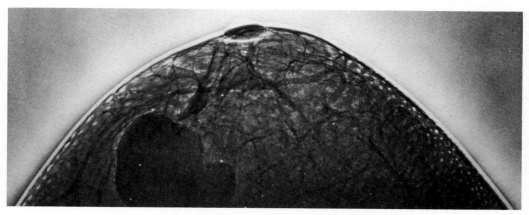

Fig. 3-50. Mamogram demonstrating fibroadenoma.

epithelial elements generally conform to a monomorphously round silhouette. There is little variability in nuclear detail from cell to cell (Fig. 3-51) and uniform spacial properties preclude molding, crowding, or other insults on distribution. Occasionally all epithelial constituents suggest an ovoid contour (Fig. 3-52), but definitive spindled stromal cells are infrequently observed.

The Scandinavian experience with fibroadenomas[20] confirms the richly cellular properties of the aspirate, but a biphasic pattern seems more characteristic with 25% of their cases featuring dissociated bipolar nuclei unsheathed of their

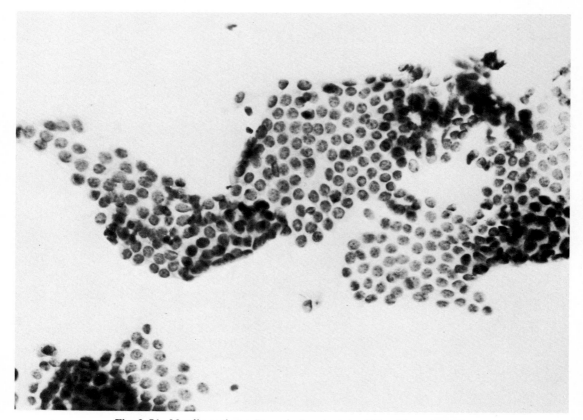

Fig. 3-51. Needle aspirate, Papanicolaou's stain, 400×, fibroadenoma.

cytoplasm. The presence of naked nuclei in aspirates with atypical cells was used as a factor to discourage an erroneous malignant diagnosis. The source of these cells was considered more likely to be from myoepithelium than stroma. The divergent appearance of naked bipolar nuclei in their series, but not in our experience could possibly be explained on the basis of differences in technique and stain, because we do not use the syringe holder and depend on manually exerted negative pressures. Nor do we use May-Grünwald-Giemsa stains routinely on air-dried material. The histological structure on which organization of the aspirated cells is predicated reflects a myriad of branching tubular ducts lined by two or three layers of regular cuboidal cells disposed in a loose fibrous matrix (Fig. 3-53).

Linsk and his associates[20] compared 210 aspirated fibroadenomas with the same number of aspirated "dysplasias" to evaluate parameters of the cellular yield and the quantity of stroma extracted. Their semiquantitative study showed

a high degree of cellularity from aspirates of fibroadenomas (67.6%) in contrast to dysplasia (3.8%) and a more generous stromal component (33.8% versus 1.9%). In our aspirates from fibrocystic disease with atypia ("dysplasias"), we found considerably fewer epithelial cells, with noticeable aberrations of nuclear properties that substantiated a suspicious diagnosis and prompted recommendation for excisional biopsy and histological study.

The aspirate of fibrocystic disease may consist of translucent semisolid material that fills the needle core, or turbid, opalescent hemorrhagic liquid that evacuates and deflates a macroscopic cyst. Direct smears and filter preparations are analyzed. The cellular population generally contains benign, uniform cuboidal cells of ductal origin in committed, communal confluence associated with foamy cells that resemble macrophages and are probably converted ductal epithelial elements (Fig. 3-54). Occasionally fibroblasts from the cyst wall are incorporated. Enlarged, polyhedral eosinophilic cells signify

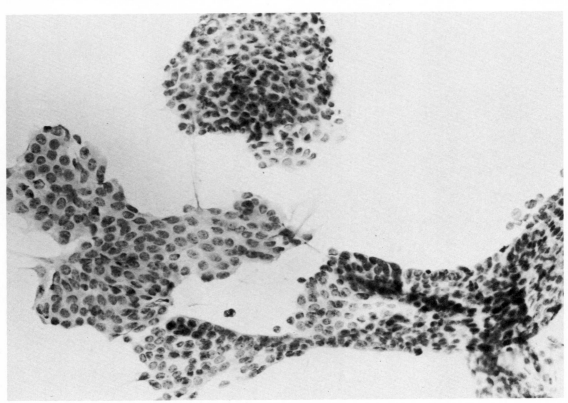

Fig. 3-52. Needle aspirate, Papanicolaou's stain, 312.5×, cytology of fibroadenoma.

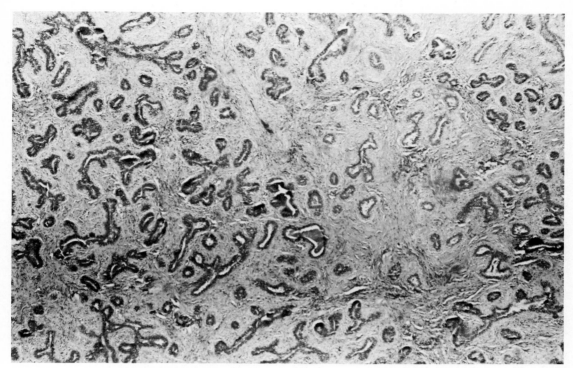

Fig. 3-53. Histological section, H&E, 50×, fibroadenoma of breast.

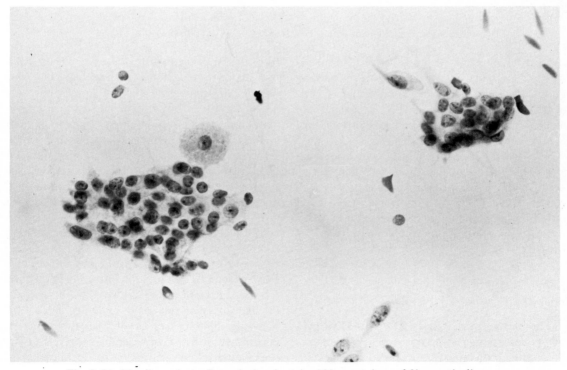

Fig. 3-54. Needle aspirate, Papanicolaou's stain, 500×, cytology of fibrocystic disease.

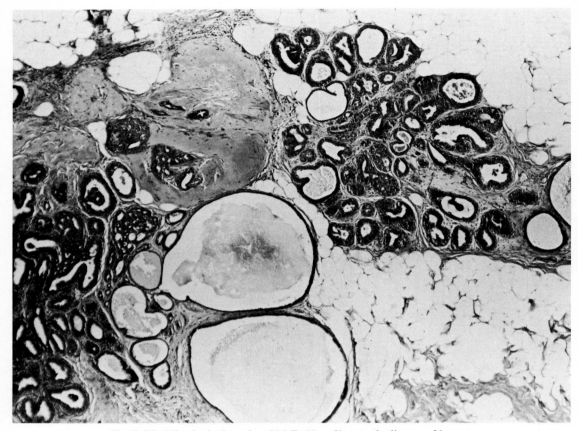

Fig. 3-55. Histological section, H&E, 50×, fibrocystic disease of breast.

apocrine metaplasia. In intraductal hyperplasia with duct ectasia (Fig. 3-55), small round cells are the frequent if not dominant cellular constituent. When dissociated cells with atypical nuclear features are comingled with this pattern, biopsy is recommended.

Sclerosing adenosis generally does not contribute a problem of cellular interpretation because the fibrous tissue restricts removal of cells, and variability in luminal size and shape of tubular aggregates helps to distinguish the lesion from differentiated or tubular carcinoma of breast.

SMEAR PROJECTIONS OF ESTROGEN-RECEPTOR ACTIVITY

The recent availability of quantitative estimates for estrogen-receptor activity in cytosol preparations of breast carcinomas has released clinical judgment about hormonal manipulation from the empirical to the objective. When positive estrogen receptors are demonstrable, the response to endocrine therapy may approach 55–60%, but a tumor with negative receptors will not regress in response to hormonal manipulation.[21] The conventional receptor assay involves quantitation by the demonstration of specific 8S and 4S binding of ^{3}H-estradiol on sucrose density gradients or segregation of nonreceptor-bound tritiated estradiol with charcoal, translated to quantitative values by Scatchard plots. The cytosol homogenate includes receptor from sources other than specific cancer cells and anatomical localization is impossible. Lee[22] developed a fluorescent estradiol conjugate for application to thick, air-dried frozen sections of mammary carcinomas and expressed the hormone binding status of the tumor as a percentage of estrogen-receptor-positive cells in the cancer cell population. Visual localization of receptor in an anatomical context was achieved,

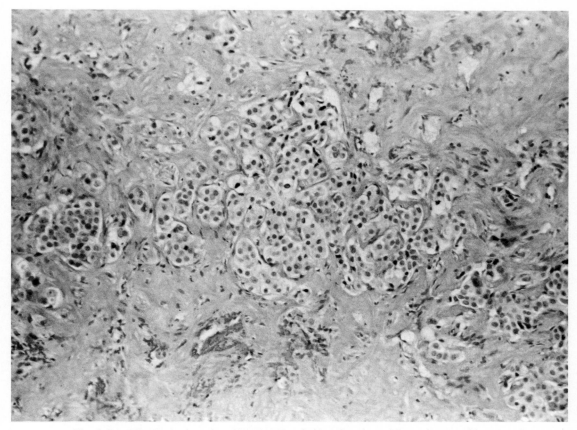

Fig. 3-56. Histological section, H&E, 160×, infiltrating duct cell carcinoma of breast.

and simultaneous demonstration of progesterone receptor was possible. These studies are in the developmental phases, but parallel statistics of the innovative histochemical method and the cytosol analysis are not yet corroborative.

In attempting to utilize Lee's method to establish a rapid slide technique for projecting receptor assay in parallel with the conventional approach performed for us by a commercial laboratory, we conceived of the possibility of utilizing the fluoresceinated conjugate for fine needle aspirate smears prepared from the same tumors as the frozen sections. We are engaged in extremely preliminary analysis of this method, and results are premature, but exciting. Figure 3-56 demonstrates the histological appearance of an infiltrating duct cell carcinoma of the breast examined by the immunofluorescent method. Frozen sections demonstrated a brilliant green fluorescence corresponding to the malignant epithelial cells (Fig. 3-57) and cytosol measure-

ments of positive proportions. The needle aspirate prepared from the same tumor (Fig. 3-58 demonstrated corresponding positive fluorescence (Fig. 3-59). We are collecting matched aspirate-frozen section couplets for comparison with chemical data, with the expectation that we can ultimately utilize the needle aspirate for a rapid prediction of hormonal response at the time the diagnosis of cancer is substantiated by needle puncture.

IDENTIFICATION OF THE METASTATIC LESION

The tendency for malignant breast epithelium to dissociate implies a potential for displacement from parent aggregates and betrayal of orderly, stationary structure. Irreverent clusters may disregard the community of the primary lesion and penetrate tissue cleavage spaces, lymphatics, or the bloodstream to colonize alien organ

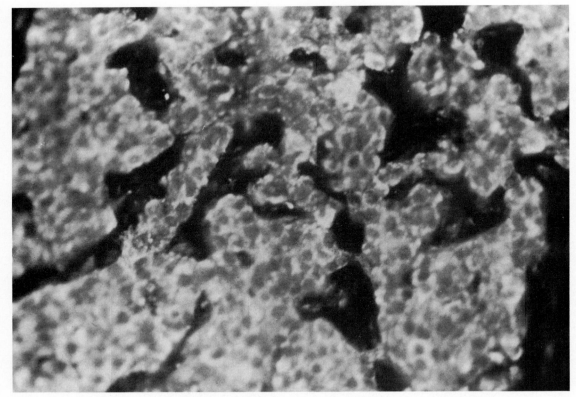

Fig. 3-57. Histological section, immunofluorescent stain demonstrating positive estrogen receptors.

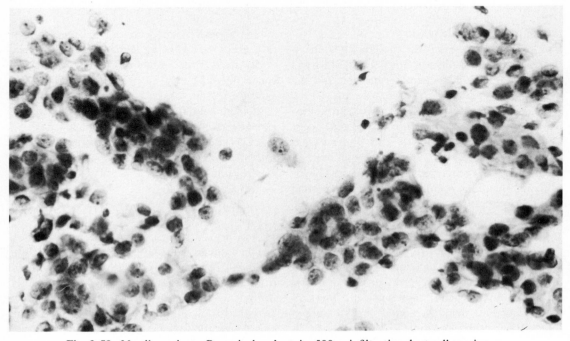

Fig. 3-58. Needle aspirate, Papanicolaou's stain, 500×, infiltrating duct cell carcinoma.

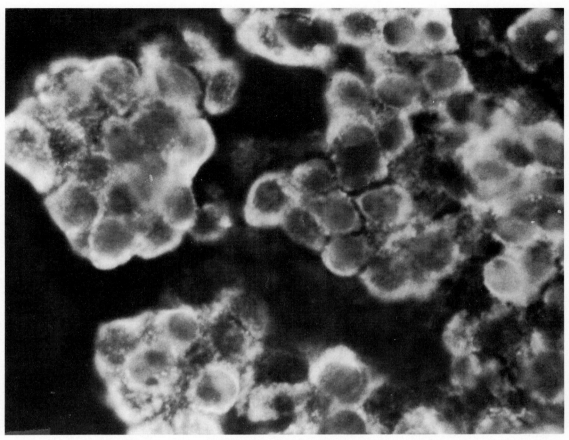

Fig. 3-59. Needle aspirate, immunofluorescent stain demonstrating positive estrogen receptors.

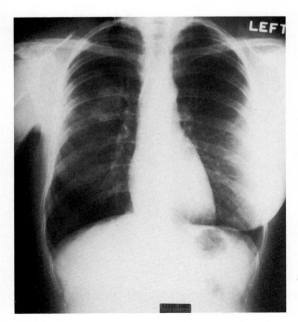

Fig. 3-60. Chest x-ray demonstrating postmastectomy appearance of metastatic lesion in right upper lobe.

systems, where residence may threaten host viability. The recognition and subsequent documentation of this process is paramount to appropriate modulation of therapy, adjustment of prognosis, modification of expectations. The aspiration biopsy is essential to a convenient, accurate, cost-effective approach to staging breast carcinoma and acknowledging its extension beyond the mammary gland.

Hepatomegaly may occur with enzymatic indications of interruption in physiological proceedings or cholestasis. Radionuclide imaging or CAT scans may demonstrate localized diminished isotopic activity or a structural defect that provides strong presumptive evidence for metastatic cancer. Verification can proceed at some risk of morbidity with a conventional core needle biopsy blindly thrust into the resisting parenchyma, or cytological validation can be accomplished by scientifically directed needle placement. The method of CAT scan directed fine needle aspiration biopsy is clarified in a separate chapter and its efficacious application is applauded.

The pulmonary metastasis suspected by clinical signs and verified by chest roentgenography can be validated by fluoroscopically directed aspiration biopsy of selected lesions. This procedure is preferable to sputum cytology because metastatic cancer cells in the lung are generally reticent to exfoliate or fail to erode into a bronchial conduit for access to the exterior. The deliberate placement of a fine needle in the preferred position assures a satisfying harvest. Figure 3-60 demonstrates the postmastectomy chest film of a 47-year-old woman who had sustained breast amputation for infiltrating duct cell carcinoma 1 year earlier (Fig. 3-61). The

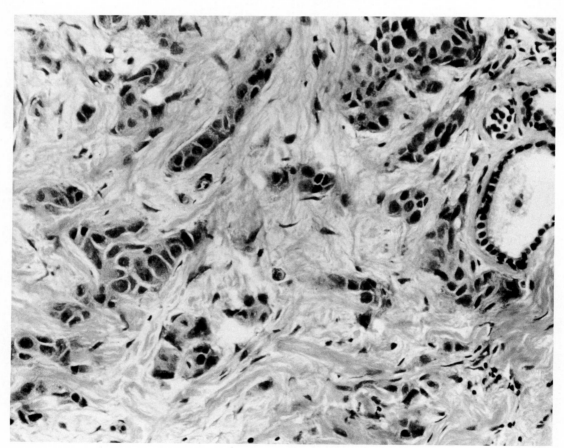

Fig. 3-61. Histological section, H&E, 315×, primary breast cancer demonstrating infiltrating duct cell carcinoma.

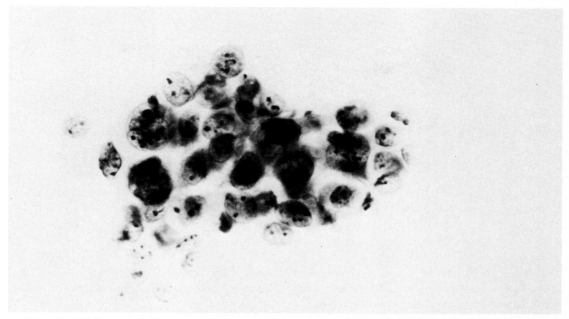

Fig. 3-62. Needle aspirate, Papanicolaou's stain, 500×, duct cell carcinoma of breast metastatic to lung.

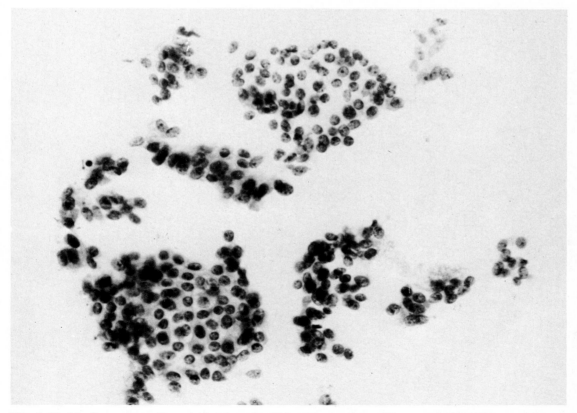

Fig. 3-63. Needle aspirate, Papanicolaou's stain, 400×, metastatic papillary carcinoma of breast involving skin.

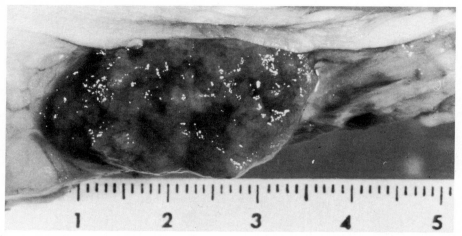

Fig. 3-64. Excisional biopsy demonstrating metastatic carcinoma involving skin.

large mass present in the right upper lobe was analyzed by aspiration biopsy and the extracted cells demonstrate nuclear characteristics of malignancy and cytological parameters that assure a glandular origin (Fig. 3-62) correlative with the histological pattern of the primary tumor. The combined systemic chemotherapeutic regimen was altered to target the pulmonary deposit.

Local recurrence in the chest wall is a frequent complaint and the cutaneous manifestations may be expressed as nodules, discrete

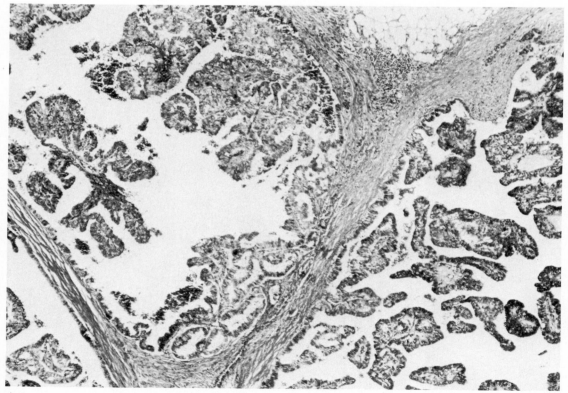

Fig. 3-65. Histological section, H&E, 62.5×, papillary configuration of breast carcinoma metastatic to skin.

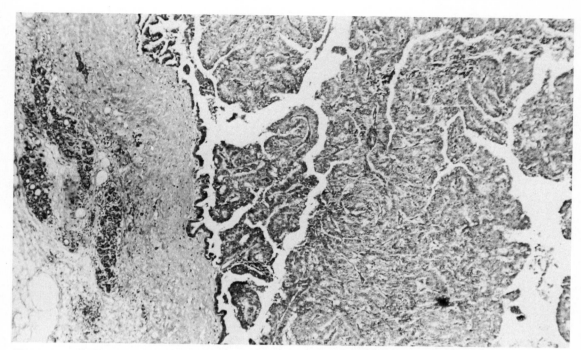

Fig. 3-66. Histological section, H&E, 62.5×, histological appearance of the primary papillary carcinoma of breast.

masses, or cirsoid aggregates conforming to dermal lymphatics. Ulcerations are less common, but may be observed if radiotherapy has been used. Figure 3-63 represents the needle aspirate from a 5 cm indurated mass that developed in the skin of the right chest wall in a 63-year-old woman. The right breast had been amputated 3 years earlier for management of papillary carcinoma. The cells are arranged in papillary clusters, and if it were not for their ectopic location in the skin and the antecedent history, it would be extremely difficult to justify

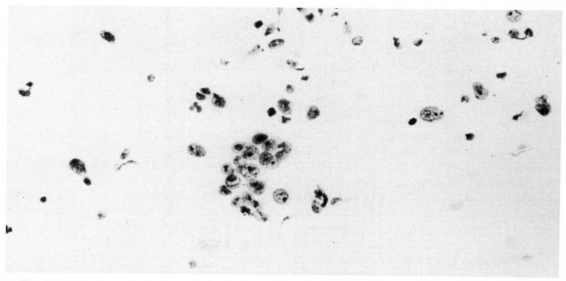

Fig. 3-67. Needle aspirate, Papanicolaou's stain, 400×, duct cell carcinoma of breast metastatic to skin.

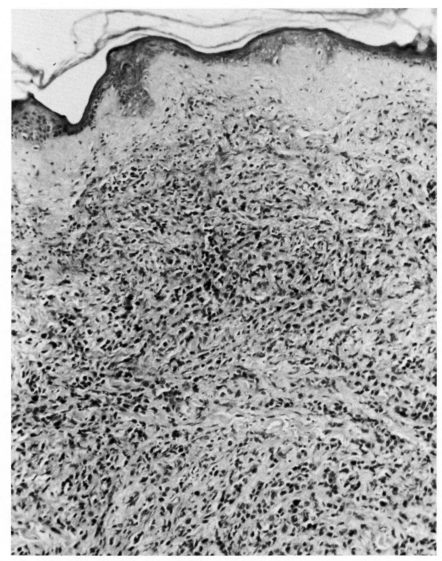

Fig. 3-68. Histological section, H & E, 160×, duct cell carcinoma metastatic to skin.

assignment of malignant criteria to the nuclei. The population is exceedingly uniform with perpetuated monotony of size and form. Nucleoli are visible but do not attract untoward attention. The assessment must predict, inclusive of all peripheral knowledge of source, history, and morphology, a well-differentiated papillary pattern. The mass was excised to achieve tumor debulking and obtain fresh tissue for hormonal receptor assays. The oval mass grew in contiguity to the skin undersurface and presented a homogeneous, red-brown, lobulated appearance without evidence for necrosis (Fig. 3-64). The confirmatory histological sections provide a distinctly papillary configuration in which several layers of regular cuboidal cells are disported on connective tissue fronds penetrated by delicate capillaries (Fig. 3-65), capitulating the papillary organization of the primary breast lesion (Fig. 3-66). Less obvious variants of skin involvement may be assessed. Figure 3-67 demonstrates small cells arranged in trabecular and linear arrays. There is variability in nuclear size but crisp envelopes are neither serrated nor convoluted. Nucleoli are prominent, variable in number, and chromatin is coarsely stippled. Skin biopsy for histological verification (Fig. 3-68) shows their arrangement in tissue in Indian file among the desmoplastic collagen fibers.

The versatility of the needle in the assessment of metastatic breast cancer is limited only by the creativity and commitment of the surveyor.

REFERENCES

1. Rimsten, A., Stenkvist, B., Johanson, H., and Lindgren, A.: The diagnostic accuracy of palpation and fine needle biopsy and an evaluation of their combined use in the diagnosis of breast lesions. *Ann Surg* **182**(1): 1–8, 1975.
2. Franzen, S., and Zajicek, J.: Aspiration biopdy in diagnosis of palpable lesions of the breast. *Acta Radiol Oncol Radiat Phys Biol* **7**(4): 241–262, 1968.
3. Kline, T. S., and Neal, H. S.: Role of needle aspiration biopsy in diagnosis of carcinoma of the breast. *Obstet Gynecol* **46**:89–92, 1975.
4. Bibbo, M., and Zuspan, F. P.: Fine-needle aspiration of the breast in an obstetrics and gynecology hospital. *Am J Obstet Gynecol* **122**(4): 525–526, 1975.
5. Frable, W. J.: Thin-needle aspiration biopsy. *Am J Clin Pathol* **65**(2): 168–182, 1976.
6. Hajdu, S. I., and Melamed, M. R.: The diagnostic value of aspiration smears. *Am J Clin Pathol* **59**(3): 350–356, 1973.
7. Kern, W. H., and Dermer, G. B.: The cytopathology of hyperplastic and neoplastic mammary duct epithelium. *Acta Cytol* **16**(2): 120–128, 1972.
8. Kreuzer, G., and Zajicek, J.: Cytologic diagnosis of mammary tumors from aspiration biopsy smears III. Studies on 200 carcinomas with false negative or doubtful cytologic reports. *Acta Cytol* **16**(3): 249–252, 1972.
9. Mouriquand, J., and Pasquier, D.: Fine needle aspiration of breast carcinoma. *Acta Cytol* **24**(2): 153–159, 1980.
10. Schondorf, H.: *Aspiration Cytology of the Breast,* W. B. Saunders, Philadelphia, 1978.
11. Fisher, E. R., Gregorio, R. M., and Fisher, B.: The pathology of invasive breast cancer. A syllabus derived from findings of the National Surgical Adjuvant Breast Project (Protocol No. 4). *Cancer* **36**(1):1–85, 1975.
12. Azzopardi, J. G.: *Problems in Breast Pathology.* W. B. Sauders, Philadelphia, 1979.
13. Ridolfi, R. L., Rosen, P. P., Port, A., Kinne, D., and Mike, V.: Medullary carcinoma of the breast. A clinico-pathologic study with 10 year follow-up. *Cancer* **40**: 1365–1385, 1977.
14. Smith, B. H., and Taylor, H. B.: The occurrence of bone and cartilage in mammary tumors. *Am J Clin Pathol* **51**(3): 610–618.
15. Griffler, R. F., and Kay, S.: Small cell carcinoma of the male mammary gland. *Am J Clin Pathol* **66**: 715–722, 1976.
16. Crichlow, R. W.: Carcinoma of the male breast. *Surg Gynec Obstret* **134**: 1011–1019, 1972.
17. Diagnostic Cytology Seminar. *Acta Cytol* **24**(2): 90–136, 1980.
18. Carstens, P. H. B., Huvos, A. G., Foote, F. W., and Ashikari, R.: Tubular carcinoma of the breast: A clinico-pathologic study of 35 cases. *Am J Clin Pathol* **58**: 231-238, 1972.
19. Fechner, R. E.: Histologic variants of infiltrating lobular carcinoma of the breast. *Hum Pathol* **6**:373–378, 1975.
20. Linsk, J., Kreuzer, G. and Zajicek, J.: Cytologic diagnosis of mammary tumors from aspiration biopsy smears II. Studies on 210 fibroadenomas and 210 cases of benign dysplasia. *Acta Cytol* **16**(2): 130–138, 1972.
21. McGuire, W. L., Horwitz, K. B., Pearson, O. H., and Segaloff, A.: Current status of estrogen and progesterone receptors in breast cancer. *Cancer* (Suppl) **39**(6): 2934–2947, 1977.
22. Lee, S. H.: Cellular estrogen and progesterone receptors in mammary carcinoma. *Am J Clin Pathol* **73**: 323–329, 1980.

Clinical Applications of Needle Aspiration Cytology in Thyroid Disease

CHAPTER

4

CELLULAR ASPECTS OF GOITER AND GRAVE'S DISEASE

Endocrine measurements, radionuclide imaging, and the clinical evaluation of the patient with thyroid disease are functions representing presumptive preoperative diagnostic data points for a clinical opinion concerning the category and extent of disease, provoking an intended therapeutic plan. The adjunctive utilization of fine needle aspiration contributes a considerably more concrete element for appraisal, a microscopic cellular representation of tissue dynamics within the gland. Needle aspiration cytology should be applied in the context of a thorough physical examination, clinical history, biochemical determinants of physiological function, and the radionuclide image. The pathologist or clinician who elects to use this procedure should accomplish a working familiarity with nuclear medicine imaging techniques. His information referable to holistic interpretation of biopsy findings must incorporate hands-on palpatory recognition of the lesion's characteristics of size, mobility, texture, multiplicity or singularity, solid or cystic character, location, fixation, and margin. He should elicit or review the history, examine the neck, and then review the nuclide silhouette of the thyroid gland (Fig. 4-1).

At our institution the patient with a palpable abnormality of thyroid structure is administered a microcurie dose of iodine-125 followed by measurements of its uptake within the gland and the subsequent distribution of the isotope to create an image of the thyroid that may be evaluated for size, symmetry, and homogeneity of isotopic distribution (Fig. 4-2). From this silhouette, the presence of single or multiple nodules and their affinity for the isotope can be demonstrated and serve as a focal point for the selection of the cellular sample (Fig. 4-3). Anatomical variants may be displayed, for example a pyramidal lobe extending from the isthmus which conceivably could be confused with the residue of the thyroglossal duct tract in the midline. The autonomously functioning "hot" nodule is considerably less often subjected to needle aspiration investigation than is the solitary "cold" nodule that carries a risk of up to 20% of harboring malignancy. A solitary lesion with diminished uptake, palpatory fluctuance, and a smooth contour can be ultrasonigraphically confirmed as cystic and the act of aspiration can serve a combined therapeutic and diagnostic function by offering opportunity for evacuation of the contents with decompression of the mass. Figure 4-4 is representative of variations in the isotopic image of the normal thyroid gland. Frame d represents a slightly oblique perspective showing the symmetry of the lobes, which are of approximately equal size, conjoined by a well-defined isthmus and composed of parenchymal tissue with uniformity of affinity for the isotope. The margins of each lobe are smoothly delineated and there is no evidence of nodular conversion. Frame g corresponds directly with the pyramidal lobe arising from the junction of the right lobe and isthmus indicated

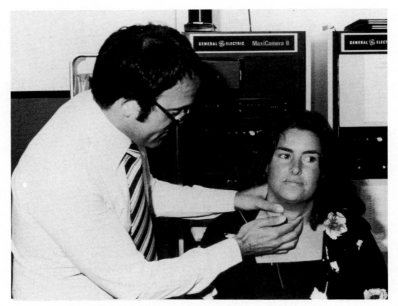

Fig. 4-1. The pathologist carefully palpates the neck prior to performing fine needle aspiration of the thyroid nodule.

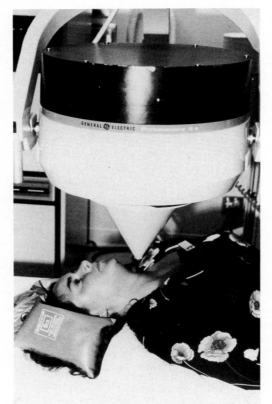

Fig. 4-2. A radionuclide scan is performed to localize the lesion and define its character, contour, and affinity for isotope.

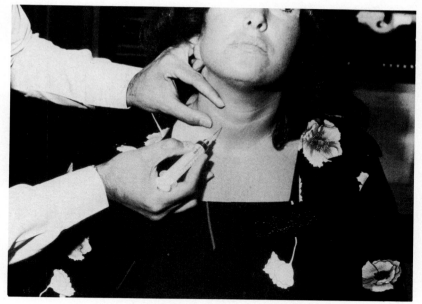

Fig. 4-3. The pathologist performs the needle aspirate.

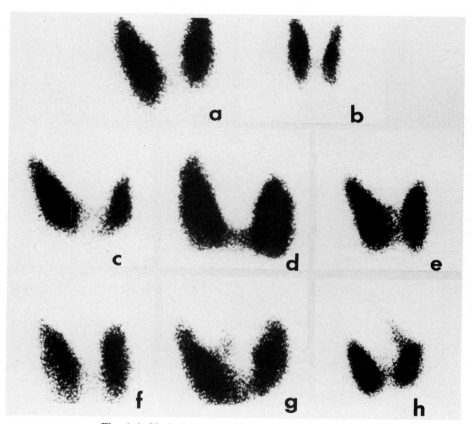

Fig. 4-4. Variations in a scintigraphic thyroid image.

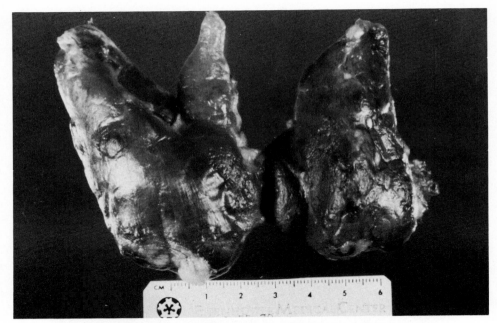

Fig. 4-5. Gross specimen, normal thyroid with pyramidal lobe.

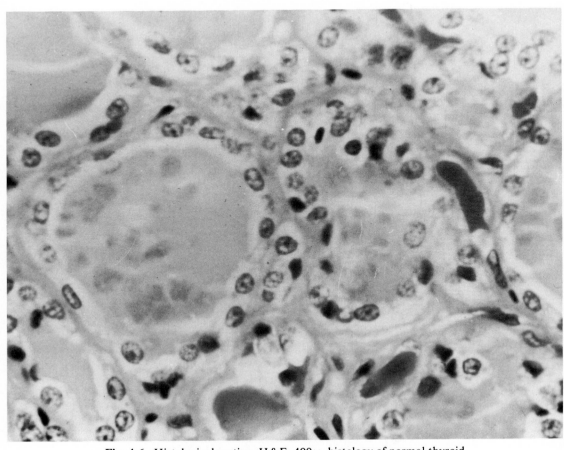

Fig. 4-6. Histological section, H&E, 400×, histology of normal thyroid.

in Figure 4-5. The penetrating needle in the area of pyramidal lobe will obtain cells indistinguishable from normal thyroid follicular elements and colloid and appropriate judgment as a normal variant should lead to the proper interpretation of the cellular sample as structurally unremarkable. The follicle cells, colloid matrix, and rarely endothelial cells are essentially the only cellular elements that should originate from aspiration of a normal gland.

Figure 4-6 demonstrates a two-dimensional histological section of normal thyroid demonstrating the juxtaposition of spheres of generally uniform size composed of uniform cuboidal cells, resting comfortably on a well-defined basement membrane, enclosing optically homogeneous, eosinophilic colloid protein, and nourished by an interlacing luxuriant capillary labyrinth penetrating small spaces between the spheres. The solid nature of the thyroid follicle should be

projected from this two-dimensional appearance. In hematoxylin-eosin preparations, the individual cells are cuboidal or low columnar and exhibit central nuclei with prominent single central nucleoli, thickened peripheral nuclear membranes without convolutionary folding, and eosinophilic cytoplasm. When these cells are transposed by the needle to a monolayer on the glass slide, fixed in ethanol, and stained by Papanicolaou's technique, their uniformity, size, and intercellular relationships are preserved, true to the tissue counterpart, with accentuation of nuclear detail by Papanicolaou's stain (Fig. 4-7). The finely stippled chromatin pattern, central nucleolus, and sharply delineated nuclear membranes are constant features of the normal follicle cells in an unstimulated posture. Note the absence of macrophages, erythrocytes, fibroblasts, or cellular aberrants in the background of the normal aspirate. Parafollicular cells that

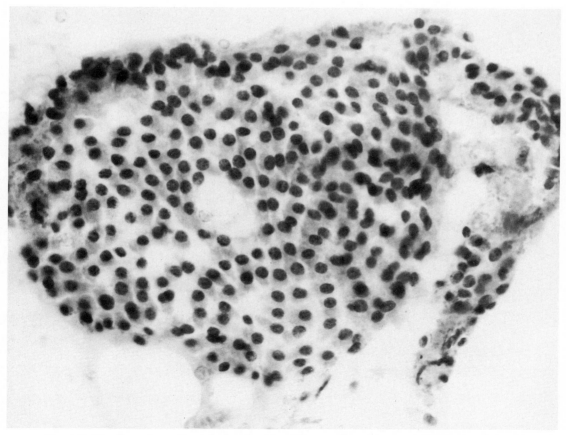

Fig. 4-7. Needle aspirate, Papanicolaou's stain, 625×, cytology of normal follicular epithelium.

produce calcitonin are not readily discernible in aspirate preparations stained by Papanicolaou's technique. This material should serve as reference for comparison studies with aberrational configurations to be discussed.

Nodular Goiter

The normal thyroid has been estimated to weigh from 8–20 gm and its parenchyma may be lobulated but is generally homogeneous and without nodularity. Thyroid weight in excess of 40 gm qualifies for a diagnosis of goiter, and benign nodular adenomatous goiter is the most frequently reported result of fine needle investigation in our experience. The patient with the nodular goiter presents with a palpably and often

visibly enlarged asymmetrical thyroid gland with variable affinity for isotope. The asymmetry and irregular distribution of isotopic activity are characteristic findings of this lesion (Fig. 4-8).

It is recommended that several punctures from various regions be obtained for adequate representation of cells from areas of different activity and structure. The thyroidectomy specimen generally presents a thinly encapsulated, bosselated, solid appearance with areas of distinct nodularity created by foci of colloid inspissation, cellular proliferation, trabecular fibrosis, variegated hemorrhage, involution, hemosiderin accumulation, and mineralization (Fig. 4-9). Despite the variegation and regional

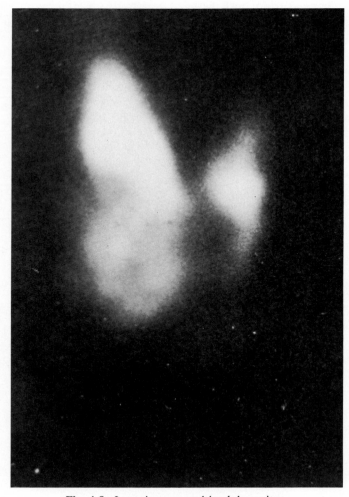

Fig. 4-8. Isotopic scan, multinodular goiter.

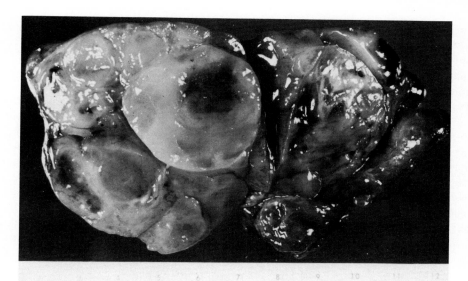

Fig. 4-9. Gross specimen, nodules of adenomatous goiter with colloid inspissation, hemorrhage, and trabecular fibrosis. ├────┤ = 1 cm.

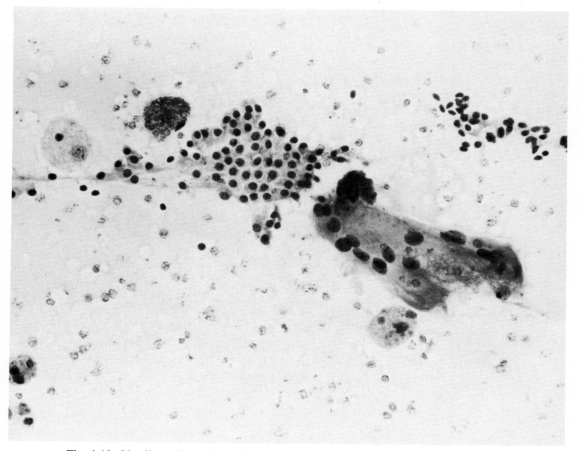

Fig. 4-10. Needle aspirate, Papanicolaou's stain, 400×, cytology of adenomatous goiter.

differences within the same lobe, the needle aspirate prepared from a predominantly solid multinodular goiter is predictably consistent in its cytological features. There are generally aggregates of uniform small cells imbricated cohesively in a tight epithelial mosaic with round nuclei that dominate cyanophilic cytoplasm, but that are organized in a regular mode of distribution. The chromatin is often homogeneously finely stippled and although some nucleoli are visible they are innocuous, round and smooth, often eccentric, and always single. These cells represent the epithelium of the colloid follicles, which physiologically iodinate and combine tyrosine molecules in the manufacture of thyroid hormones, encompassing the thyroglobulin storage matrix within the interior of the spheres created by their arrangement. Seen in juxtaposition are large cyanophilic cells with granular cytoplasm and eccentric, regular reniform nuclei with prominent nucleoli representing macrophages that usually contain phagocytosed hemosiderin representing the mineral residue from antecedent episodes of intraparenchymal hemorrhage (Fig. 4-10, 4-11).

Fragments of optically homogeneous eosinophilic colloid matrix may represent mechanical dislodgement by the aspirate or follicular disruption in a sequential proliferative-involutional response to thyroid-stimulating hormone (TSH). Although follicle cell aggregates and hemosiderin-in-laden macrophages must be present by definition, other elements, including erythrocytes, fibroblasts, foamy histiocytes, collagen, and incontinent colloid may be observed in the needle aspirate. This variegated cytological pattern may reflect the multiplicity of histological components observed in tissue preparations of the nodules (Fig. 4-12) in which there are combinations of follicles of variable size and colloid content created by variable numbers of follicle cells separated by interstitial edema, hemorrhage, trabecular fibrosis, organizing cholesterol deposits, incontinent hemosiderin, necrosis, focal cellular proliferative activity or cyst formation. This aberration is apparently the result of alter-

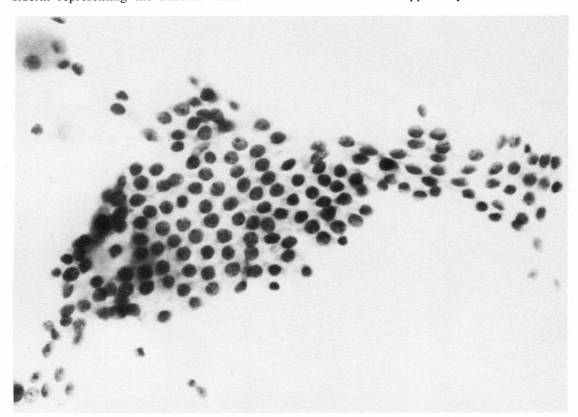

Fig. 4-11. Needle aspirate, Papanicolaou's stain, 625×, cytology of adenomatous goiter.

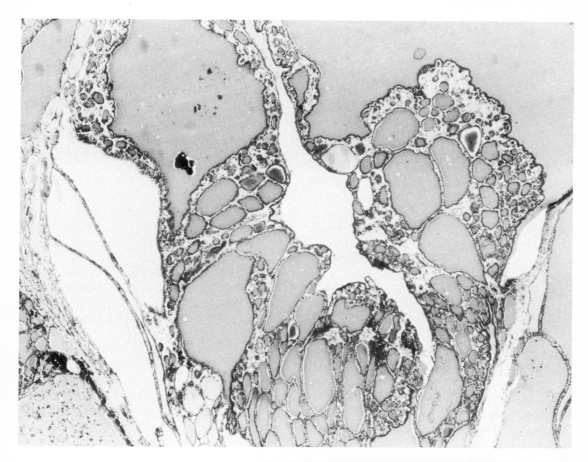

Fig. 4-12. Histological section, H&E, 80×, adenomatous goiter.

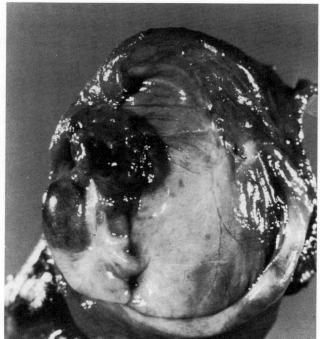

Fig. 4-13. Gross specimen, evacuated cystic adenomatous nodule.

nating proliferative and involutional response to TSH stimulation of multifactorial etiology[1] that may be related to goitrogens and results in thyroid enlargement and defined multinodularity. In our experience, the follicular epithelial component is generally well preserved when it originates from solid nodules and that variations in nuclear size and shape, disturbances in nuclear cytoplasmic ratios, and other clues to malignant transformation or dysplasia are not generally seen. When the nodules are primarily cystic (Fig. 4-13), the evacuated fluid contains cells that have been suspended in a liquid medium, deprived of vascular nourishment. They therefore appear less cohesively integrated and nuclear detail is less sharply focused with chromatin blurring, an expected change.

Aspirates prepared from cystic lesions generally contain a larger number of foamy and hemosiderin-laden macrophages (Fig. 4-14) in association with microfollicles encapsulating colloid, which have been released from the cyst wall into the internal bath (Fig. 4-15). The ultrasonographically substantiated cystic nodule should first be examined with a 22-gauge needle to establish the presence of internal fluid but a second puncture may be performed with an 18- or 20-gauge needle for purposes of evacuation and decom-

pression. It is possible, however, that the larger core needle may induce additional bleeding.

The management of cystic lesions by conservative methods, that is, evacuation of fluid and cytological estimation of the absence of malignant cells, must be modulated by the information that cystic lesions can harbor malignancy. Three of 15 malignancies evaluated by Wallfish et al.[2] were partially or completely cystic and two of these demonstrated an ultrasonically mixed picture. Einhorn and Franzen[3] reported histologically verified malignancy in 2 of 61 cases in which the aspiration biopsy showed cystic lesions, and this figure could be spuriously low because only 22 cases actually came to operation.

Acceptable guidelines for management of the cystic lesion relate to the size of the lesion and recurrence of hemorrhagic cyst fluid after repeated aspiration. If the cyst is small, evacuation results in total collapse, the cytological content is benign, the ultrasonographic scan reflects an entirely cystic rather than mixed picture, and there is only one recurrence leading to repeated aspiration, the lesion can be treated conservatively.[2] If the size of the lesion exceeds 4 cm, there are frequent and multiple recurrences, cytological atypia or evidence for malignancy,

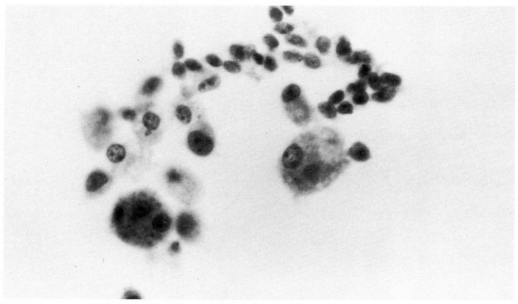

Fig. 4-14. Needle aspirate, Papanicolaou's stain, 625×, hemosiderin-laden macrophages and reactive follicular epithelial cells in cyst fluid.

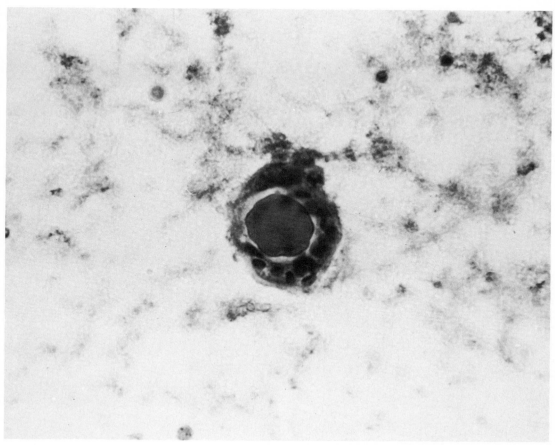

Fig. 4-15. Needle aspirate, Papanicolaou's stain, 625×, dissociated follicle with central colloid in cyst fluid.

and a mixed ultrasonic pattern, the lesion should be excised and subjected to thorough histological study. Although Crile and Hawk[4] advocate the installation of a sclerosing agent, we have not recommended this to our clinicians in order to avoid masking the spontaneous tendency of the lesion to recur and thereby signal necessity for further intervention. Whether the cyst is considered *de novo* or a degradative phenomenon in pre-existent goiter, the cellular constituency and histopathology are the same (Fig. 4-16). However, cystic conversion of an adenoma should produce a monomorphous pattern and a malignancy should yield cells that are generally discernible.

Papillary Hyperplasia (Grave's Disease)

The cytomorphological presentation of papillary hyperplasia, or Grave's disease, in fine needle aspirations has received little attention in the literature and well-delineated characteristics have not been formulated, probably because the clinical appearance, biochemical data, and response to therapy are so characteristic that histoarchitectural studies are not mandated for initiation of therapy, (Fig. 4-17). Thyroid tissue is available for study in postoperative situations in which a medical regimen has not induced complete involution and the histological pattern generally reflects inefficient medical control. Because of this limitation in clinical acquisition, cytological examples that we include are the result of direct specimen sampling. The cells are projected *en face* as a cohesive and intricate mosaic of uniform epithelial cells that appear considerably more succulent than unstimulated normal follicular variants (Fig. 4-18). Cytoplasm is abundant, nuclei are evenly distributed, and cellular boundaries, although indistinct, are

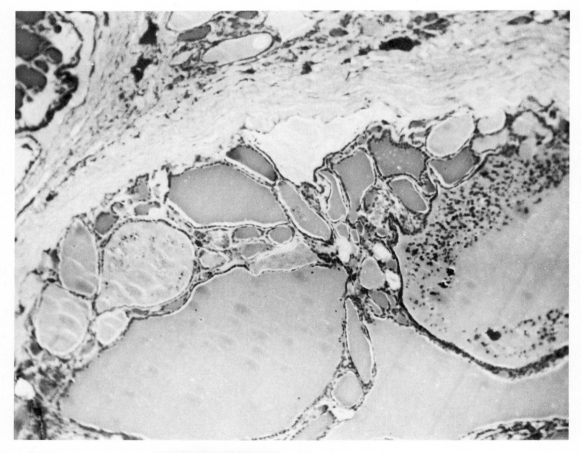

Fig. 4-16. Histological section, H&E, 125×, cyst wall with changes of adenomatous thyroid.

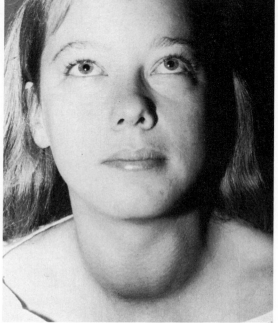

Fig. 4-17. Diffuse thyroid enlargement and exophthalmus of Grave's disease.

detectable. The projected impression is reminiscent of tall columnar cells of endocervical origin as they appear in a honey-combed mosaic. Careful search denotes the presence of definitive papillary conformations (Fig. 4-19) and the most striking characteristic is the absolutely uniform distribution of nuclei around the periphery of the papillation. This is in contradistinction to the appearance of cells from papillary carcinoma in which nuclear molding, arbitrary orientation of long axes with respect to basement membrane, crowding, and ground-glass clearing or vacuolization are evident. The nucleoli of these cellular elements are prominent as an expression of accelerated physiological function.

In some areas there are abortive attempts at follicular organization. Inflammatory cells, macrophages, oncocytic elements, and extravasated blood are conspicuously absent. The cellular sample from Grave's disease is generally monomorphous and nonvariegated in correlative loyalty to the gross appearance in which the entire gland is diffusely involved by the same process and the transected surface appears lobulated and plethoric or manifests a pale tan pallor (Fig. 4-20). This is in contradistinction to the variegated multinodular goiter that releases a multiplicity of cell types as its cellular representative. There is identity established between the papillary aggregation of the individual cells as projected in cytological specimens and in the two-dimensional histological configuration where the papilla is composed of a delicate, vascularized connective tissue stalk supporting uniform and well-palisaded surface epithelial cells (Figs. 4-21, 4-22). Despite this limited information concerning the cytology of Grave's disease, these cellular features in concert with

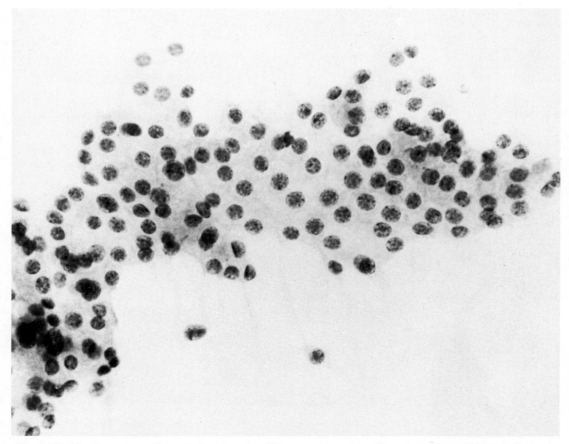

Fig. 4-18. Needle aspirate, Papanicolaou's stain, 625×, cytology of papillary hyperplasia (Grave's disease).

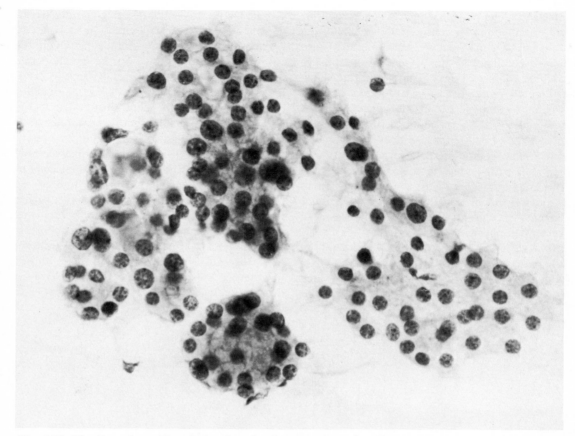

Fig. 4-19. Needle aspirate, Papanicolaou's stain, 625×, cytology of papillary hyperplasia (Grave's disease).

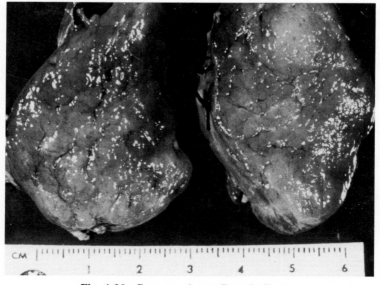

Fig. 4-20. Gross specimen, Grave's disease.

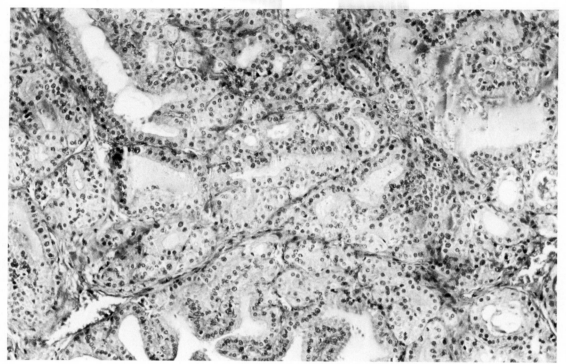

Fig. 4-21. Histological section, H&E, 160×, papillary hyperplasia (Grave's disease).

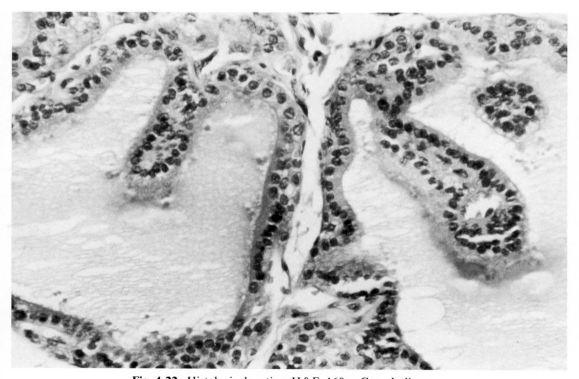

Fig. 4-22. Histological section, H&E, 160×, Grave's disease.

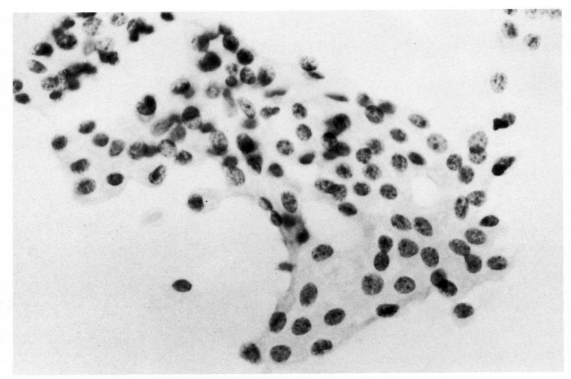

Fig. 4-23. Needle aspirate, Papanicolaou's stain, 625×, follicular adenoma.

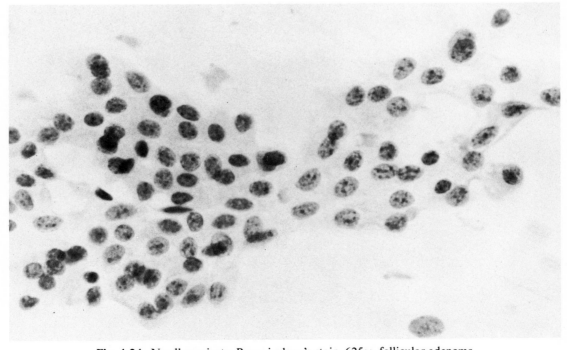

Fig. 4-24. Needle aspirate, Papanicolaou's stain, 625×, follicular adenoma.

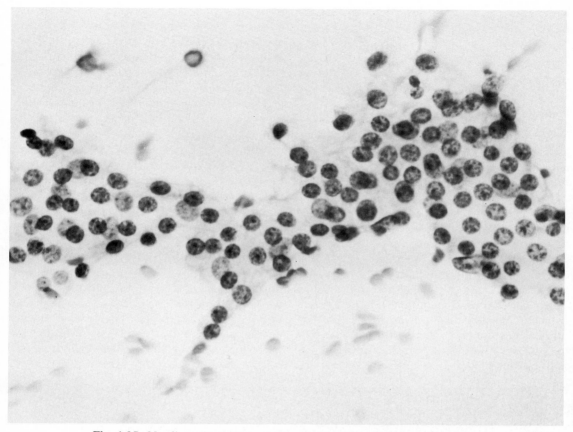

Fig. 4-25. Needle aspirate, Papanicolaou's stain, 625×, follicular adenoma.

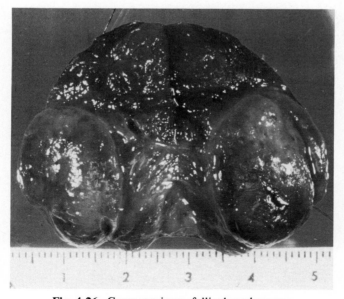

Fig. 4-26. Gross specimen, follicular adenoma.

biochemical and clinical evidence substantiate the diagnosis.

INVASIVE HARVEST FROM THE SOLITARY NODULE

Follicular Adenoma

The frequency of follicular adenoma in our aspiration experience follows that of adenomatous goiter and thyroiditis. The diagnosis is substantiated by histological confirmation that a solitary nodule, delineated by a specified capsule from surrounding compressed thyroid parenchyma is composed of a uniform cell type different from extracapsular tissue, which does not exhibit aggressive intent to violate the capsule or penetrate the lumen of blood vessels within its substance.[5] The diagnosis of follicular adenoma and its differentiation from well-differentiated follicular carcinoma resides in the surgical microscopist's demonstration histologically of the absence of capsular and angioinvasion, a decision that requires conscientious inspection of the entire periphery of the lesion. Vascular elastic connective tissue stains are necessary to identify angioinvasion that may not be clearly recognizable from the hematoxylineosin preparations. The cellular composition of the follicular adenoma by definition is uniform and generally monotonous and in the follicular type there is definitive arrangement around luminal spaces to recapitulate normal follicular appearances (Figs. 4-23, 4-24). Although there may be slight anisokaryosis, the nuclear characteristics are generally recapitulated throughout all cellular components of the aspirate and may be characterized by sharply delineated nuclear envelopes, coarse chromatin stippling, prominent chromocenters, and abundant granular cyanophilic cytoplasm. In some instances the cells are organized in sheets (Fig. 4-25). In contradistinction to the experience of Lowhagen and Spenger[6] we did not observe the presence of macrophages in any of our histologically proved adenomas and, in fact, reserved the presence of histiocytes to implicate the nodules of adenomatous goiter. Colloid may be invariably present and appears

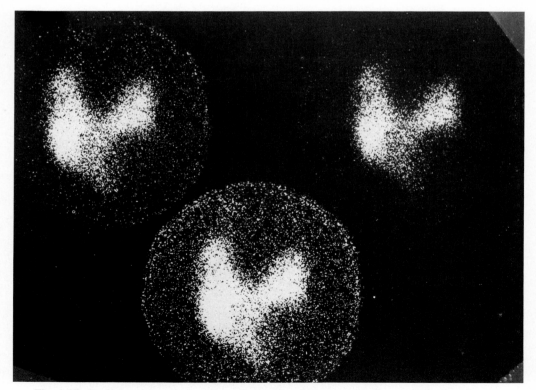

Fig. 4-27. Radioisotopic scan demonstrating cold nodule corresponding to follicular adenoma.

optically homogeneous, eosinophilic, and somewhat stellate in its deposition. The nodule from which the cells are derived is usually solid, homogeneous, minimally variegated but may be modified by hemorrhage, cystic degeneration, or compression necrosis (Fig. 4-26). The nodule correlates scintigraphically with deprivation of radionuclide activity, manifesting as a solitary cold nodule (Fig. 4-27). Microscopically, a dense collagenous connective tissue capsule envelopes a cellular proliferation of follicle cells arranged around luminal spaces of variable size often creating a mixed macro- and microfollicular pattern with trabecular coalescence (Fig. 4-28). Examination of the entire capsule for invasion is negative and special stains fail to disclose the presence of angioinvasion. The identification of the lesion by fine needle aspiration as a follicular adenoma must carry with it the medicolegal disclaimer that the technique is limited to differ-

entiate this lesion from well-differentiated follicular carcinoma. What the preoperative evaluation of the nodule by this method achieves, however, is an opportune operative plan to perform hemithyroidectomy to provide tissue for histological examination of the total tumor.

The next case demonstrates emphatically why the cellular sample is not accurately predictive of the biological behavior of the lesion it represents. The tumor presented as a solitary cold nodule in the lower pole of the left thyroid lobe of a 41-year-old male (Fig. 4-29). The lesion was well delimited, thinly encapsulated, homogeneous and viable without evidence of necrosis, cystic degeneration, or hemorrhage. The needle aspirate produced a uniform population of cells with minimal variability in size, shape, or chromatin dispersion. Orientation was regular, cytoplasm abundant, and the general appearance quite innocuous (Fig. 4-30). Histological sec-

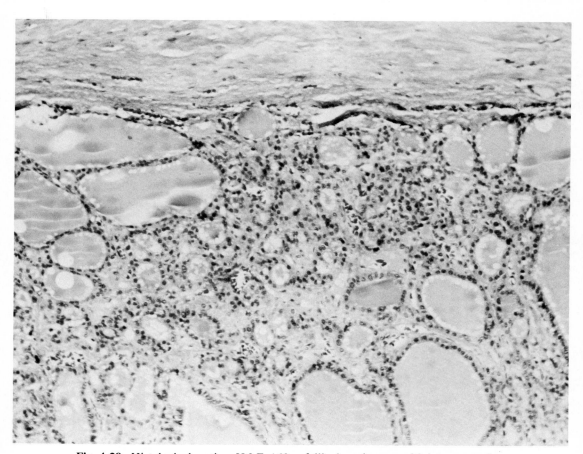

Fig. 4-28. Histological section, H&E, 160×, follicular adenoma with intact capsule.

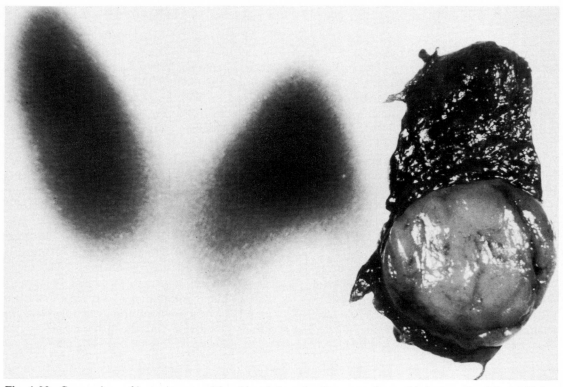

Fig. 4-29. Comparison of isotopic scan with cold nodule and solitary neoplasm at inferior pole of thyroid lobe.

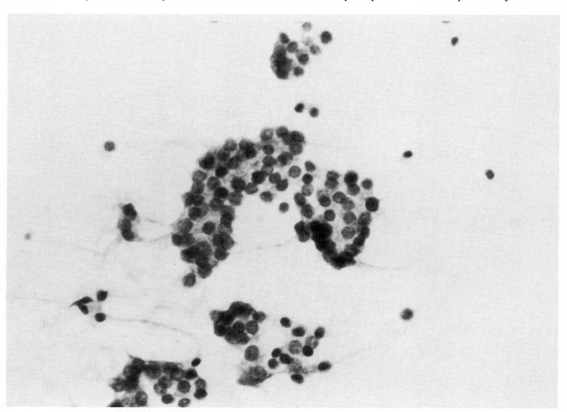

Fig. 4-30. Needle aspirate, Papanicolaou's stain, 625×, bland, uniform follicular cells.

tions demonstrated a trabecular arrangement of uniform cells without a follicular organization but with propagation through the capsule where the collagenous fibers were obliterated and the neoplastic cells interfaced with adjacent colloid parenchyma (Fig. 4-31). A closer perspective on this area of invasion emphasized the monotony of the individual cells as an incongruity to their penetrative capability (Fig. 4-32). Small nests of similar bland cells were present within endothelially lined vascular spaces constituting microangioinvasion (Fig. 4-33). Therefore cytomorphological detail is not reliable in predicting the inherent biological capabilities of a follicular lesion but can only verify the presence of a follicular neoplasm. This caveat is clearly emphasized in the work of Lowhagen, et al.[6,7]

FOLLICULAR CARCINOMA

In contradistinction to the delineated or encapsulated nodule with metastatic potential, the invasive follicular carcinoma that intrudes into adjacent parenchyma without definitive interface may propagate a cell with characteristic malignant features that make its recognition more than tentative. Figure 4-34 demonstrates the aspirate from such a lesion, implicating variability in nuclear size, shape, and distribution with coarse hyperchromasia, focal attempts at nuclear molding, and little tendency for follicular arrangement. In this instance the cytology is predictive of a malignant element but follicular organization is not immediately transparent despite the well-defined follicles of variable size, close juxtaposition, and invasive nests characteristic of the parent lesion (Fig. 4-35). Another example of the overtly malignant follicular neoplasm (Fig. 4-36) discloses anaplastic nuclei with probosci, irregular convolutionary folding of the envelopes, chromatin blurring nucleolar prominence, chromatin gossameric network, and definitive follicular arrangement. Marked variability in nuclear size with organization faithful to the follicular arrangement makes a benign consideration untenable (Fig. 4-37). The neo-

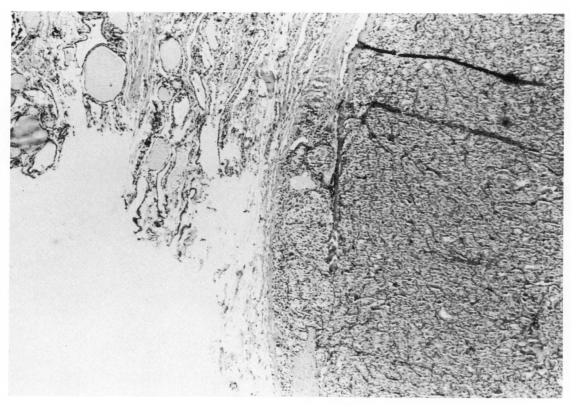

Fig. 4-31. Histological section, H&E, 80×, extension of follicular epithelium through capsule.

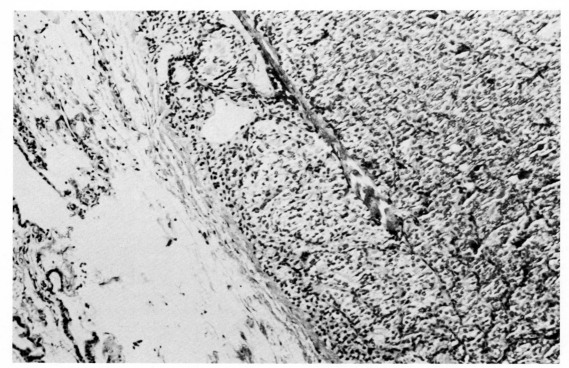

Fig. 4-32. Histological section, H&E, 160×, extension of follicular epithelium through capsule.

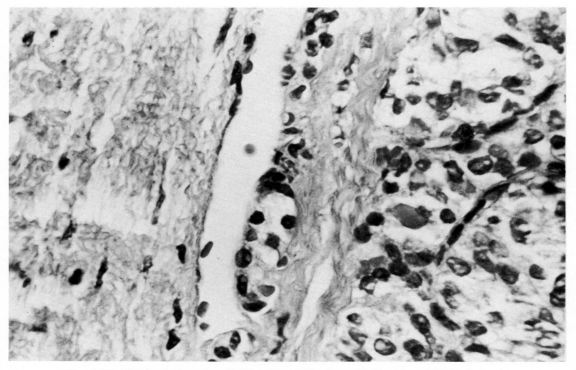

Fig. 4-33. Histological section, H&E, 400×, follicular epithelium in small blood vessel.

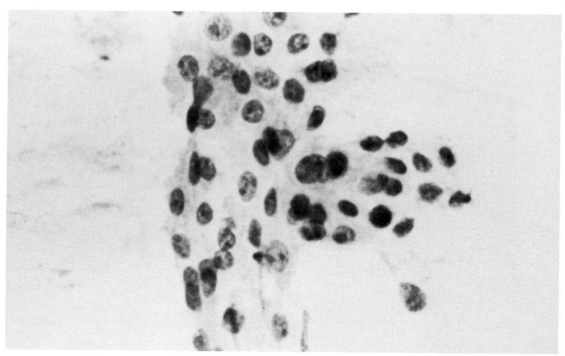

Fig. 4-34. Needle aspirate, Papanicolaou's stain, 400×, follicular carcinoma.

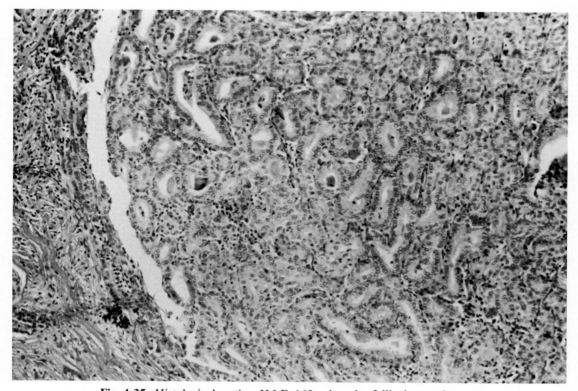

Fig. 4-35. Histological section, H&E, 160×, invasive follicular carcinoma.

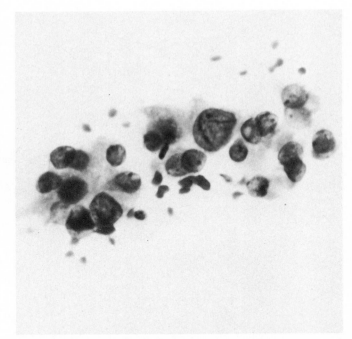

Fig. 4-36. Needle aspirate, Papanicolaou's stain, 625×, follicular carcinoma.

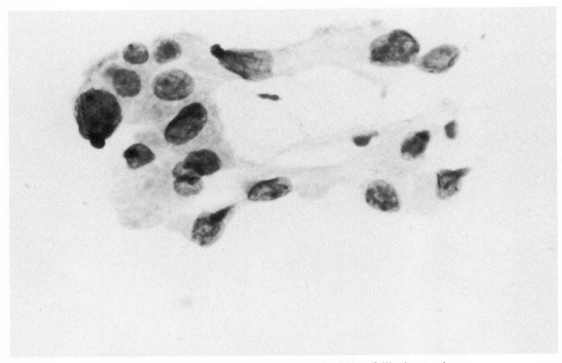

Fig. 4-37. Needle aspirate, Papanicolaou's stain, 800×, follicular carcinoma.

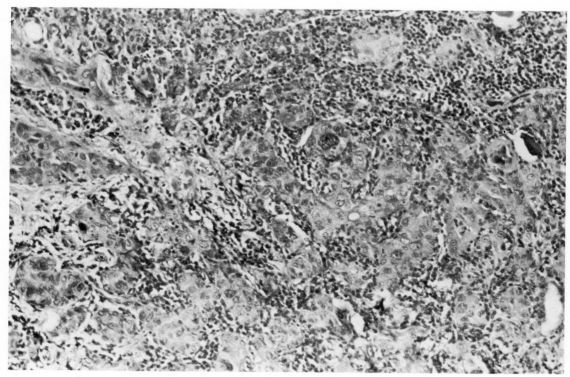

Fig. 4-38. Histological section, H&E, 160×, follicular carcinoma.

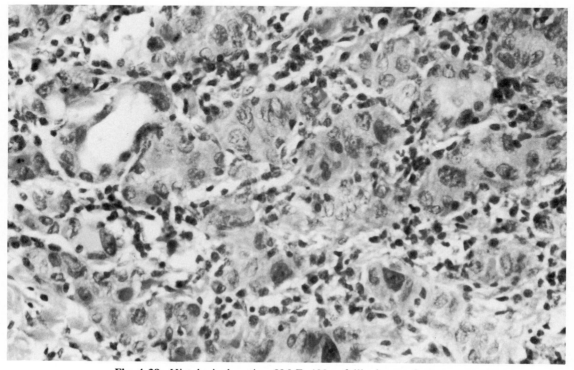

Fig. 4-39. Histological section, H&E, 400×, follicular carcinoma.

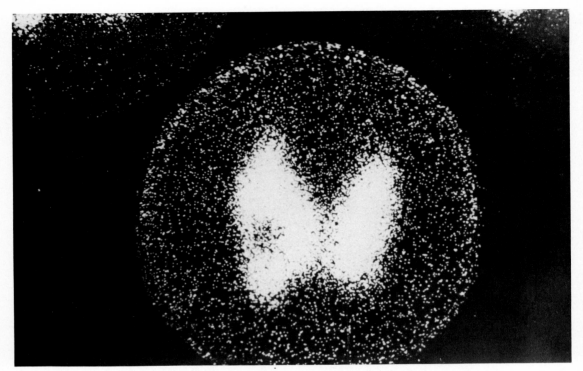

Fig. 4-40. Radioisotopic scan demonstrating a cold nodule in the right thyroid lobe.

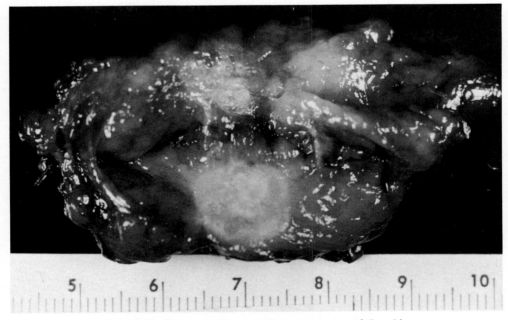

Fig. 4-41. Gross specimen, papillary carcinoma of thyroid.

plasm in its histological posture is composed of cells identical to those in the cytological preparation arranged in trabecular aggregates and microfollicles. The same nuclear aberrations are clearly represented, despite differences in fixation and stain (Figs. 4-38, 4-39). The value to the surgeon of predicting this lesion preoperatively is the justification for his decision to proceed with total thyroidectomy and a preoperative search for metastases through hematogenous avenues.

PAPILLARY CARCINOMA

Papillary carcinoma is the most frequently encountered malignancy of the thyroid gland at our institution. The lesion presents as an unencapsulated, often sclerotic cold nodule (Figs. 4-40, 4-41). The aspirate is generally cellular and the cells relate in papillary configurations. Although the cells are cohesive, respecting community affiliation, there is disregard for regimentation resulting in arbitrary alignment, postures of oblique repose, crowding, and overpopulation. The categories of nuclear aberrations have been described. Most commonly is a ground-glass vesicularity that is peculiar to all nuclei, despite subtleties in shape variation due to convolutional differences in nuclear membranes (Fig. 4-42). When a delicate fibrovascular core is incorporated into the cellular aggregate, the papillary architecture is unequivocal, but generally the papillary structure is hinted rather than concretely replicated in the cell sample. There is essentially no disparity between the cytological appearance of the nuclei in the

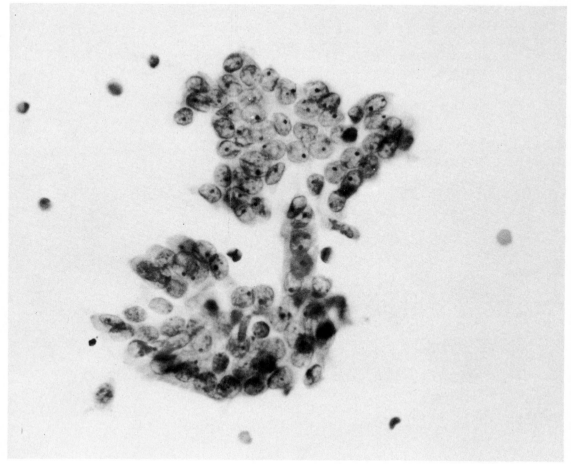

Fig. 4-42. Needle aspirate, Papanicolaou's stain, 800×, papillary carcinoma of thyroid.

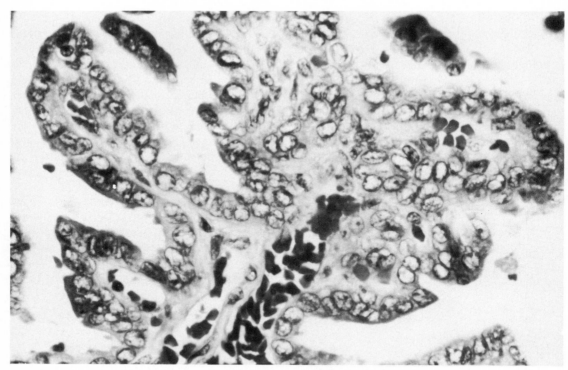

Fig. 4-43. Histological section, H&E, 625×, papillary carcinoma of thyroid.

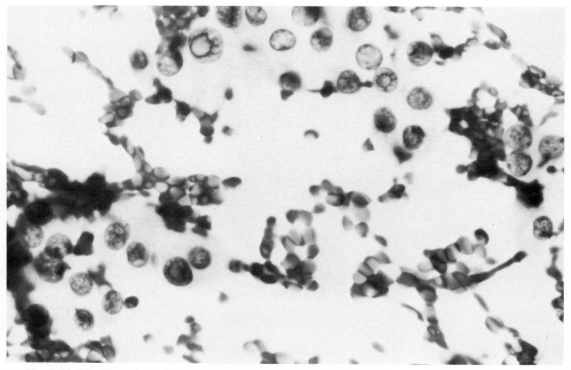

Fig. 4-44. Needle aspirate, Papanicolaou's stain, 800×, intranuclear inclusions of papillary carcinoma.

Papanicolaou-stained needle aspirate preparation and in the histological section (Fig. 4-43). The nuclear morphology of papillary carcinoma of the thyroid reported by Gray and Doniach[8] incorporated the concept of vesicular clearing, the empty quality of the indented nuclei, and frequent dissociation with follicular arrangements that permit a differentiation from the epithelial changes of papillary hyperplasia. Their ultrastructural studies described cytoplasmic invaginations of nuclei implicated as pseudoinclusions but this antedated Hapke and Dehner's[9] recent appellation as the "Orphan Annie nucleus," which they emphasized to be a reliable indicator of papillary carcinoma of the thyroid when present as a diffuse change in tissue preparations from a thyroid neoplasm. They cautioned, however, that this is not pathognomonic of papillary carcinoma because it has been identified in biologically proved follicular carcinoma and in one case each of diffuse hyperplasia and follicular adenoma.

This variant of papillary carcinoma is demonstrated in Figure 4-44, representing a clinical aspirate from a solitary cold nodule at the inferior pole of the right lobe in a 49-year-old male (Fig. 4-45). This cellular harvest consisted of polyhedral cells of variable size, arranged in pseudopapillary clusters and characterized by the presence of abundant cyanophilic cytoplasm with delineated margins. Many of the nuclei exhibited crisply defined, usually eccentrically oriented, optically clear or opalescent vacuoles marginated by condensed homogeneous chromatin that accentuated the nucleolemma. Uniform clearing or ground-glass change of the entire nucleus was not seen, although some of the vacuoles assumed a stippled pattern. Although nuclei varied considerably in size, there was subtle poikilokaryosis. Psammoma bodies were not identified in the Papanicolaou-stained material. Concordance with the papillary nature of the neoplasm in its histological projection, with establishment of identity discloses the absence of disparate features (Fig. 4-46). Psammoma bodies were present within the vascularized stroma of individual papillations (Fig. 4-47) but were retained within the tissue despite evacuative effort. Certainly their presence in association with pseudopapillary aggregates would

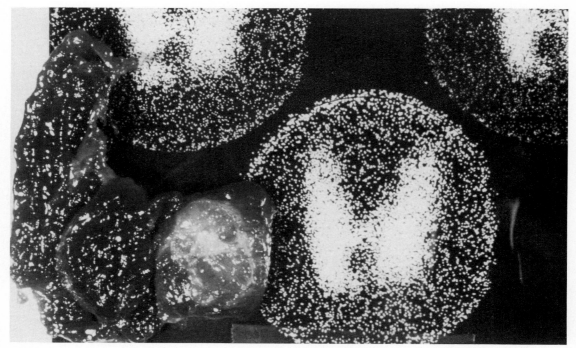

Fig. 4-45. Comparison of cold nodule, junction of right lobe and isthmus with gross specimen demonstrating follicular carcinoma.

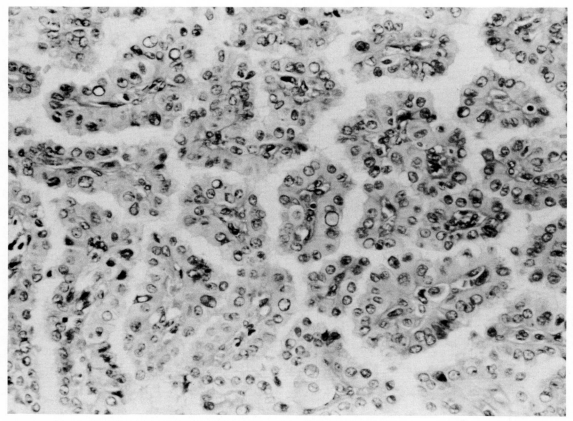

Fig. 4-46. Histological section, H&E, 400×, papillary carcinoma with intranuclear vacuoles.

provide unequivocal evidence of a papillary neoplasm of the thyroid.

The same lesion demonstrated an additional finding of clinical relevance, consisting of the aggregation of cells with polyhedral silhouette and intranuclear vacuoles in a definitive follicular and trabecular arrangement (Fig. 4-48). The follicular attitude was not predicted from the needle aspirate but there is concordance in nuclear detail. This feature supports the postulate advanced by Chen and Rosai[10] that a follicular variant of papillary carcinoma exists and may constitute the dominant or exclusive pattern of the nodule. The presence of intranuclear vacuoles in a predominantly follicular lesion could predict that the behavior will correspond to that of a papillary tumor with indolent growth, intrathyroidal metastases, and lymph node involvement rather than aggressive dissemination to bones, viscera, and other patterns of dissemination associated with follicular carci-

noma. The appearance of these nuclear changes was attributed to fixation and tissue processing, because clear nuclei were not observed on frozen sections or on tissue imprints.

By the technique that we use in our laboratory, a monolayer of fresh cells obtained by needle aspiration with rapid fixation in 95% ethanol and application of Papanicolaou's stain resulted in the demonstration of clear or ground-glass intranuclear vacuoles that correlated directly with tissue findings in both the papillary and follicular phases. In the cytological preparation the entire nucleus was not involved, since a rim of preserved homogeneous cytoplasm circumscribed the clear or ground-glass space that presented as the vacuole. In the corresponding tissue preparations, virtually the entire nucleus was involved by the alteration that extended to the nuclear membrane. The mechanism for the delineation or formation of such vacuolar spaces is not elucidated by the observation that ethanol-

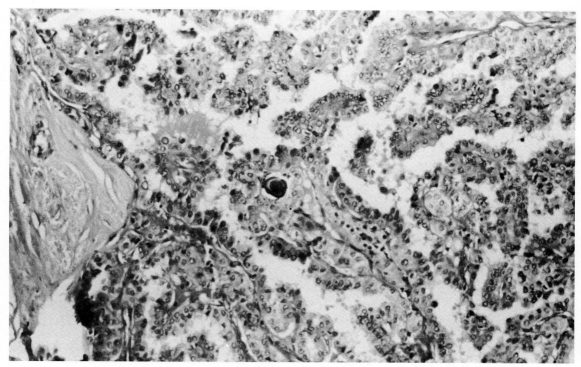

Fig. 4-47. Histological section, H&E, 160×, papillary carcinoma with psammoma body.

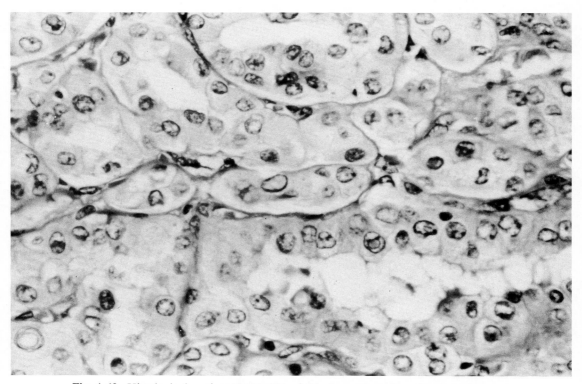

Fig. 4-48. Histological section, H&E, 625x, follicular variant of papillary carcinoma.

fixed, Papanicolaou-stained material will demonstrate these nuclear features. However, since the demonstration does not appear to be a function of a specific fixation or staining method, it is quite possible that they are the result of intranuclear cytoplasmic invaginations, as indicated in 1968 by the electron microscopic studies previously mentioned.[8] This case, called attention[11] to the concept that Papanicolaou's stain may demonstrate nuclear clearing or vacuoles correlative with comparable tissue changes in histologically defineable papillary and follicular carcinoma, contributing an intriguing cellular feature for the discerning cytopathologist. The absence of hemosiderin-laden macrophages, normal follicle cells, or other contaminant cellular elements must also be emphasized.

ANAPLASTIC OR UNUSUAL LESIONS

Medullary Carcinoma

Our experience with the aspirate appearance of medullary carcinoma of the thyroid is limited to two cases that occurred in a 3-year period of study, the infrequency of which reflects the relatively unusual incidence of this tumor, which constitutes from 3–10% of all thyroid cancers. The lesion is cytomorphologically and biopotentially peculiar because of the inconsistency of its cellular constituents and because as a malignant tumor it remains sufficiently differentiated to produce calcitonin, serotonin, prostaglandins,[12] and generally amyloid, which can be detectable in Papanicolaou-stained preparations as extracellular, optically homogeneous, cyanophilic, birefringent extracellular droplets with apple green irridescence under polarized light. When the cytological appearance is nonspecific, the presence of amyloid, corroborated by alkaline Congo red stains isolates the category of tumor to which the biopsy must be assigned. The parent cell of origin is the parafollicular or C cell of the thyroid, which is not apparently recognizable in Papanicolaou-stained preparations, although there are appropriate descriptions for May-Grünwald-Giemsa alternatives.[13] The parafollicular cell does not engage in the *gestalt* of the follicular sphere but is present in the interfollicular space and remains separated from the thyroglobulin, assuming no responsibility for its production.

The patients are generally male, may present peculiarly with diarrhea, and may be involved in a familial constellation of endocrinopathy, the common denominator of which is a cell capable of amine precursor uptake and decarboxylation (APUD system) eventuating in the simultaneous development of pheochromocytomas, neural ectodermal lesions, and the evolution of the multiple endocrine adenomatosis syndrome. Prognosis is guarded, despite the sometimes indolent proliferative effort.

The two common cytological presentations of medullary carcinoma of the thyroid are represented by our case material.

A 47-year-old female presented with a history of a persistent left cervical mass that slowly increased in size, eventuating in tracheal pressure but without production of significant

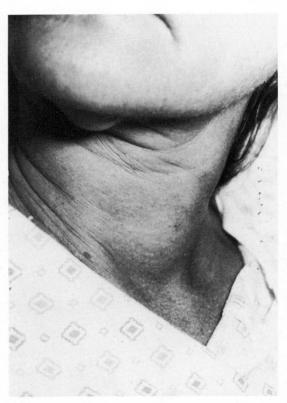

Fig. 4-49. Clinically enlarged thyroid and adjacent lymphadenopathy.

cosmetic deformity (Fig. 4-49). A thyroid scan demonstrated significantly diminished radionuclide activity involving virtually the superior two-thirds of the left lobe (Fig. 4-50). A preoperative aspirate from the lymph node in the anterior triangle adjacent to the left lobe was productive of a luxuriantly cellular sample in which the individual elements appeared definitively spindled with a loosely cohesive tendency to fascicular formation. The cytoplasm appeared very slightly granular, gently tapering to points of extinguishment (Figs. 4-51, 4-52). The nuclei were usually fusiform, slightly indented with prominent nucleoli and gently stippled chromatin. Nuclear molding, anaplasia, and mitoses were not identified.

An aspirate from the left thyroid lobe contained singly disposted cells that were either triangular or polyhedral or recapitulated the spindle cell quantity of the nodal metastasis (Fig. 4-53). Amyloid stains were not performed because the diagnosis of medullary carcinoma

was not cytologically or clinically suspect until the availability of the histological preparations. The cyanophilic, homogeneous, irregularly stellate deposits compatible with amyloid were not identified, but amyloid was reported in only 64% of the cases of Sodersterom et al.[13] in which they reviewed aspirated material from 18 patients with medullary carcinoma of thyroid. The resected thyroid lobe was completely replaced by a homogeneous, slightly granular, densely indurated neoplasm that preserved only a thin peripheral rim of compressed thyroid parenchyma (Fig. 4-54). The histological sections demonstrated rather bland-appearing spindle cells arranged in tightly cohesive whorled fascicles in a milieu of collagenosis (Fig. 4-55) with obliterative propagation arbitrarily sparing residual follicles of variable size, barely recognizable histologically as thyroid derivatives. Focal areas of eosinophilic homogenization in the stromal matrix corresponded to birefringent green areas under polarization microscopy. Postopera-

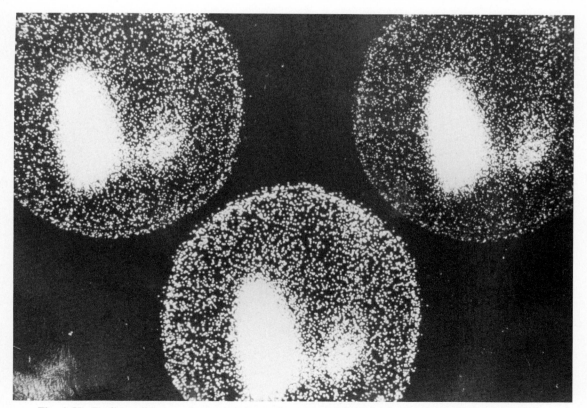

Fig. 4-50. Radionuclide scan demonstrating replacement of the left lobe by an extensive cold nodule.

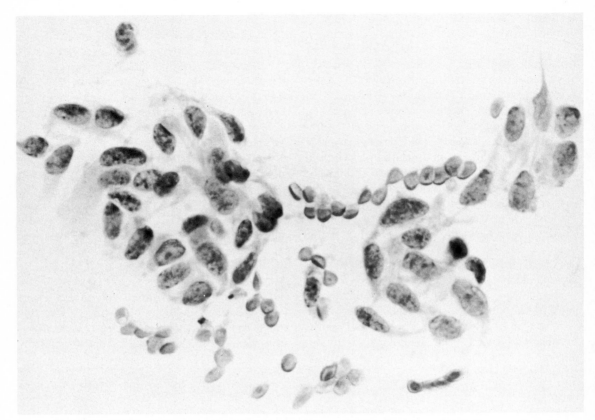

Fig. 4-51. Needle aspirate, Papanicolaou's stain, 800×, spindle cell variant of medullary carcinoma.

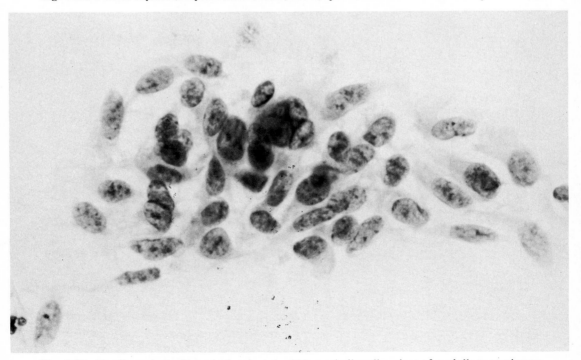

Fig. 4-52. Needle aspirate, Papanicolaou's stain, 800×, spindle cell variant of medullary carcinoma.

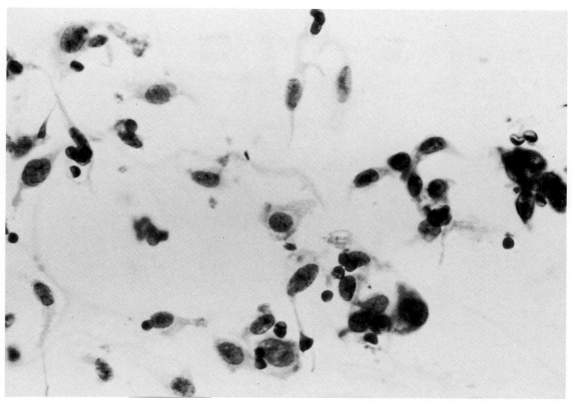

Fig. 4-53. Needle aspirate, Papanicolaou's stain, spindle cell variant of medullary carcinoma.

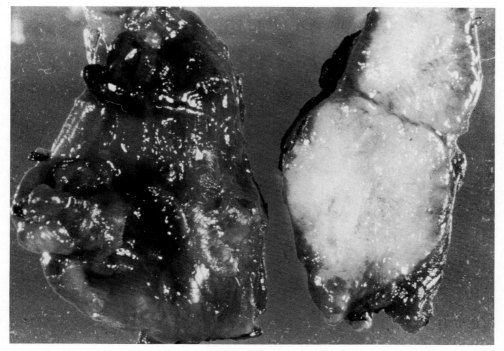

Fig. 4-54. Gross specimen, extensive replacement of left thyroid lobe by homogeneous gray-white tumor.

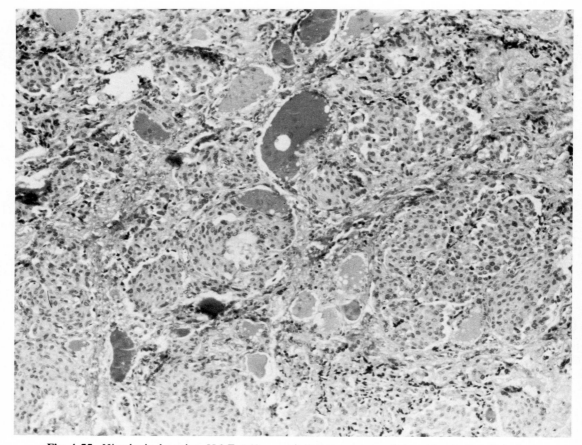

Fig. 4-55. Histological section, H & E, 160×, medullary carcinoma of thyroid, spindle cell variant.

tively the serum calcitonin level was ascertained at 6000 pg% and the history of persistent diarrhea was elicited. In addition, the patient admitted that a sibling was under investigation for a cold thyroid nodule.

The second patient was a 29-year-old female who presented with a palpable cold thyroid nodule and cervical lymphadenopathy. An aspirate prepared from her thyroid lobectomy presented congeries of small cells with densely hyperchromatic nuclei, minimal cytoplasm, and an essentially undifferentiated quality (Fig. 4-56 and 4-57). Amyloid was deposited in characteristic form. Her tumor was characterized by sheets of small cells often arranged in linear concentric whorls reminiscent of the pattern of infiltrating lobular carcinoma of breast (Fig. 4-58). Apple green birefringent amyloid deposits were noted in the stroma and in cellular cytoplasm.

It is impossible to verify the red granules

described by Sodersterom et al.[13] and the Ljunberg[14] in their descriptions of derivatives of medullary carcinoma stained by the May-Grünwald-Giemsa technique because we do not use this medium nor do we examine air-dried preparations that may have manipulated the contour of the medullary carcinoma cells to be characteristically triangular, as described by the Scandinavians. The spindle cell variant should represent a clue to this diagnosis and appropriate investigative procedures should be initiated when spindle cells appear in aspirates from the thyroid or adjacent lymph nodes. Frable has recorded a case similar to ours and Corwin[12] implicates the spindle pattern as a discrete variant of medullary carcinoma and refers to Williams, who related the spindle cell pattern to a poor prognosis. In the case of medullary carcinoma of the thyroid of familial incidence, needle aspiration cytology offers a useful adjunctive tool for evaluating members of the family in

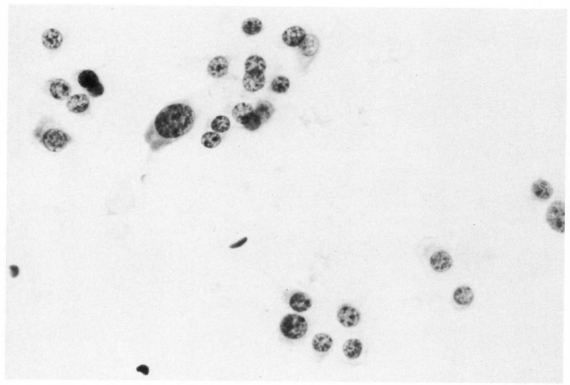

Fig. 4-56. Needle aspirate, Papanicolaou's stain, 800×, small cell variant of medullary carcinoma.

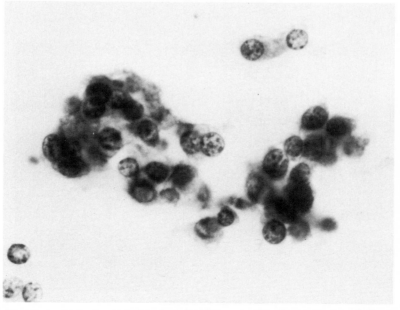

Fig. 4-57. Needle aspirate, Papanicolaou's stain, 800×, small cell variant of medullary carcinoma.

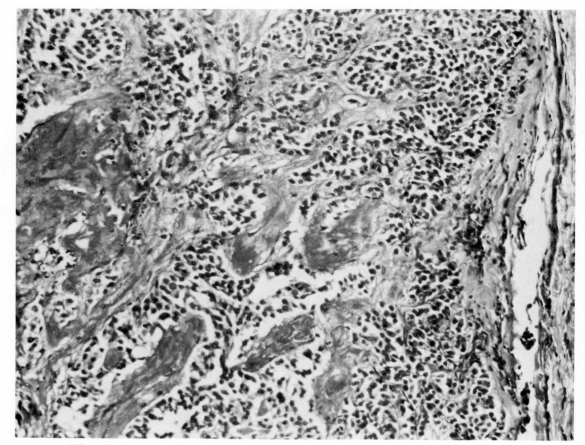

Fig. 4-58. Histological section, H&E, 200×, medullary carcinoma with amyloid stroma.

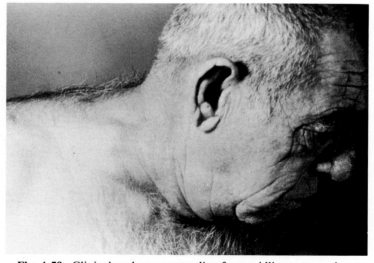

Fig. 4-59. Clinical neck mass extending from midline to trapezius.

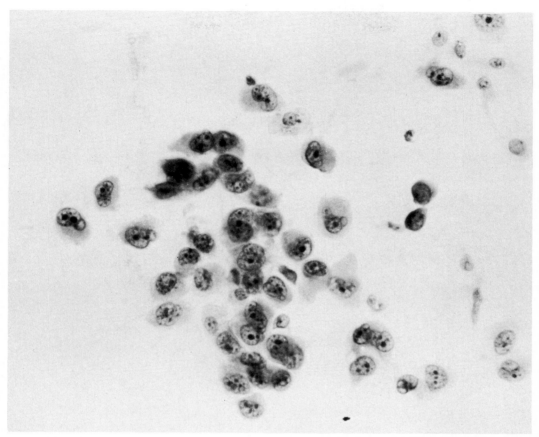

Fig. 4-60. Needle aspirate, Papanicolaou's stain, 500×, cytology of large cell anaplastic carcinoma of thyroid.

whom serum calcitonin radioimmunoassay studies complemented by thyroid scintigraphic imaging may indicate the presence of thyroidal lesions requiring immediate investigation.

Anaplastic Lesions

Giant cell carcinoma of the thyroid is considered one of the most aggressive neoplasms in man.[15] Its etiology has been variably related to TSH, radioiodine therapy, external radiation, and transformation from differentiated thyroid cancer. The tumor develops in the elderly and the victim is generally dead within 6 months to a year, with a mean survival time of 2.5–4.0 months. Therapy should be planned as if the patient had disseminated disease at the outset and may include surgery, chemotherapy, and radiation, but the results are invariably inconsequential, with death supervening rapidly.

The needle aspiration biopsy can establish the diagnosis and spare the elderly patient surgery, particularly if he is at risk because of medical problems or because tumor progression contraindicates surgical intervention. We have had one spectacular opportunity to study the cytology of giant cell carcinoma of the thyroid by this method. The patient was an 80-year-old male who presented with a 3-months' history of a mass in the neck that extended from the midline laterally to the trapezius (Fig. 4-59). Cough, hoarseness, and allergic rhinitis were present. The mass was examined by needle puncture without local anesthesia and was not painful. The cells consisted of giant polyhedral epithelial elements with coarsely serrated nuclear envelopes, vesicular chromatin, and prominent nucleoli (Fig. 4-60) with an occasional tendency to spindling. Glandular formations, keratinized cells, and papillary formations were not seen.

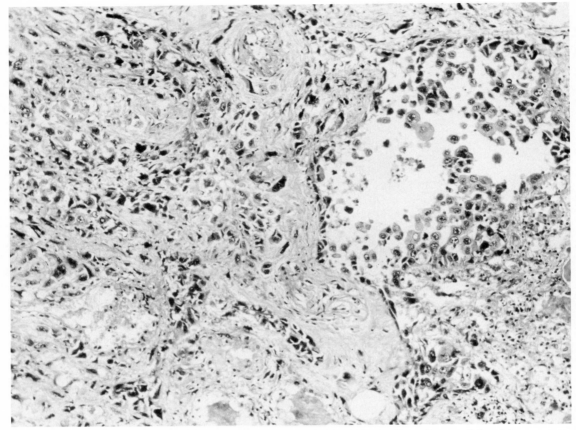

Fig. 4-61. Histological section, H&E, 200×, anaplastic large cell carcinoma of thyroid.

A cytological diagnosis of large cell anaplastic carcinoma of thyroid provoked radiotherapy, but the patient deteriorated rapidly with progressive disease. The necropsy examination 4 months following diagnosis demonstrated extensive involvement of the neck, mediastinum, and lungs by tumor. Microscopic sections disclosed replacement of thyroid parenchyma by sheets and acinar arrangements of large, anaplastic epithelial cells (Fig. 4-61) comparable to the cytological population. Transition from thyroid follicles in which colloid was observed as residual, optically homogeneous eosinophilic substance was noted, but antecedent differentiated carcinoma was not documented. The differential diagnosis includes squamous cell carcinoma primary in the thyroid, but the distinction proves academic because the ultimate course of both lesions is fatal.

We have not had the opportunity to examine small cell undifferentiated carcinoma of the thyroid by this technique because of its rarity in our particular patient population. Despite the controversy concerning the progenitor cell for this lesion, there is morphological confusion between lymphoma and small cell undifferentiated carcinoma in tissue sections, and this conceivably could be perpetuated in a cytological medium. Aldinger et al.[15] state unequivocally that small cell undifferentiated carcinomas of the thyroid are in actuality lymphomas and therefore radiosensitive, so the distinction may not be relevant.

THE MEDICAL BIOPSY: THYROIDITIS

The definitive work in the cytological diagnosis of thyroiditis is the Scandinavian experience,[16] which is overwhelmingly comprehensive

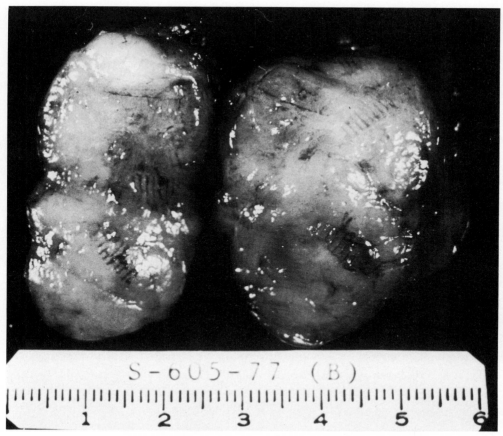

Fig. 4-62. Gross specimen, Hashimoto's thyroiditis.

and complete. The value of needle aspiration cytology in the community hospital evaluation of the patient with presumptive thyroiditis is to obviate surgery if a cytological population characteristic for thyroiditis correlates with antibody titers indicative of Hashimoto's type or provides a cellular prototype of another specific inflammatory lesion. Nonspecific thyroiditis is suggested by a luxuriant harvest of lymphocytes in a monomorphous population. Hashimoto's thyroiditis characteristically and by definition universally affects the entire thyroid (Fig. 4-62) so that puncture at any arbitrary location should provide the cells for pattern recognition, and these must include oncocytic follicular cells (Hürthle cells), plasma cells, lymphocytes, and even cellular detritus from the immunological degradation in progress (Fig. 4-63). This corresponds to intense plasma cell and lymphocytic infiltration of thyroid parenchyma with follicle formation and development of germinal centers in association with Hürthle cell change, cellular necrosis (Fig. 4-64), and the appearance of anti-thyroglobulin antibodies. In subacute thyroiditis, which may be virally induced, the thyroid may be segmentally involved in contradistinction to the Hashimoto's type, and a dense gray-white infiltrate may replace the lobules of the normal lobe (Fig. 4-65). The isolation of multinucleated histiocytes in association with lymphocytes (Fig. 4-66) is a clue to the diagnosis of de Quervain's thyroiditis in which granulomas form in the interstitial matrix of the thyroid with follicular destruction and replacement. Multinucleated histiocytes, epithelioid histiocytes, and lymphocytes may congregate in circumscribed, lamellated foci to create classical granulomas (Fig. 4-67). When the surgeons develop trust in the diagnostic capability of the procedure for predicting thyroiditis, tissue follow-up declines,

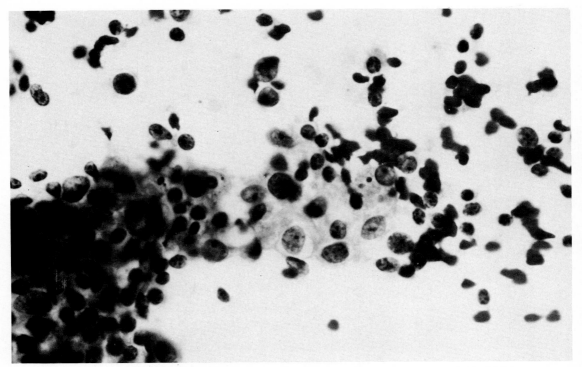

Fig. 4-63. Needle aspirate, Papanicolaou's stain, 625×, cytology of Hashimoto's thyroiditis.

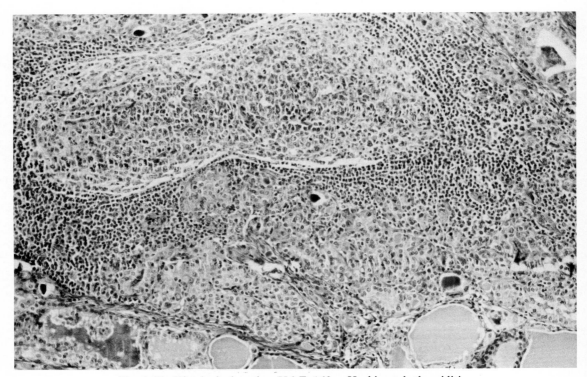

Fig. 4-64. Histological section, H&E, 160×, Hashimoto's thyroiditis.

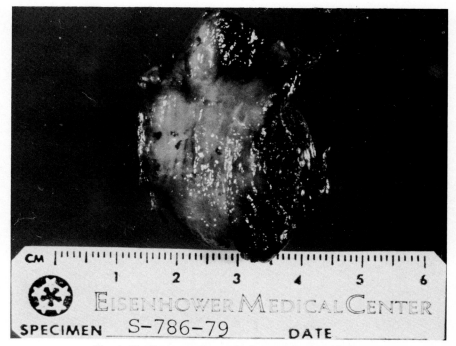

Fig. 4-65. Gross specimen, de Quervain's thyroiditis.

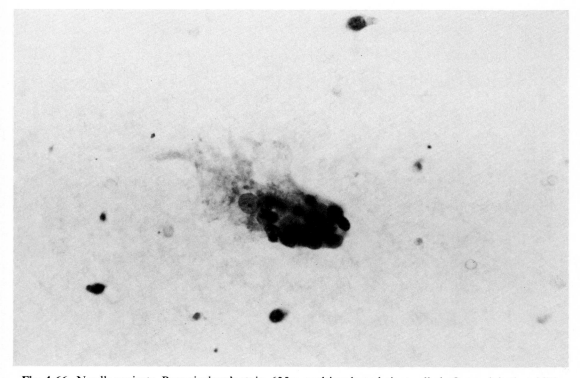

Fig. 4-66. Needle aspirate, Papanicolaou's stain, 625×, multinucleated giant cell, de Quervain's thyroiditis.

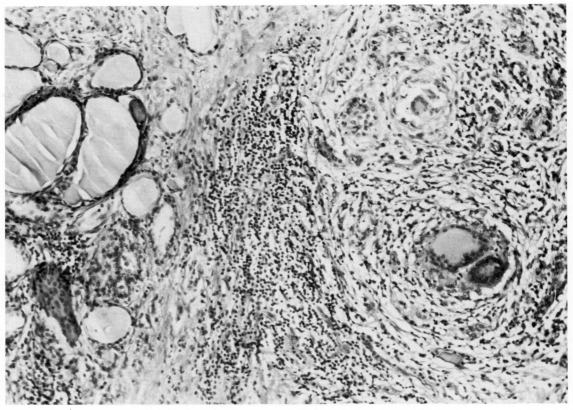

Fig. 4-67. Histological section, H&E, 160×, de Quervain's thyroiditis.

but the patient benefits by the repeal of surgical referral.

REFERENCES

1. Werner, S. C., and Ingbar, S. H., Eds.: *The Thyroid,* 3rd ed. Harper & Row, New York, 1971.
2. Walfish, P. G., Hazani, E., Strawbridge, H. T. G., Miskin, M., and Rosen, I. B.: A prospective study of combined ultrasonography and needle aspiration biopsy in the assessment of the hypofunctioning thyroid nodule. *Surgery* 82(4): 474–482, 1977.
3. Einhorn, J., and Franzen, S.: Thin needle biopsy in the diagnosis of thyroid disease. *Acta Radiol* 58(5): 321–336, 1962.
4. Crile, G., and Hawk, W. A.: Aspiration biopsy of thyroid nodules. *Surg Gynecol Obstet* 136: 241–245, 1973.
5. Meissner, W. A., and Warren, S.: Tumors of the thyroid. AFIP Fascicle Number Four, Second Series, 1968.
6. Lowhagen, T., and Sprenger, E.: Cytologic presentation of thyroid tumors in aspiration biopsy smear. *Acta Cytol* 18(3): 192–197, 1974.
7. Lowhagen, T., Granberg, P. O., Lundell, G., Skinnari, P., Sundblad, R., and Willems, J. S.: Aspiration biopsy cytology in nodules of the thyroid gland suspected to be malignant. *Surg Clin North Am* 59(1): 3–18, 1979.
8. Gray, A., and Doniach, I.: Morphology of the nuclei of papillary carcinoma of the thyroid. *Br J Cancer* 23(1): 49–51, 1968.
9. Hapke, M. R., and Dehner, P.: The optically clear nucleus, a reliable sign of papillary carcinoma of the thyroid? *Am J Surg Pathol* 3: 31–38, 1979.
10. Chen, T. K., and Rosai, J.: Follicular variant of thyroid papillary carcinoma; a clinicopathologic study of six cases. *Am J Surg Pathol* 1: 123–130, 1977.
11. Kaminsky, D. B.: The intranuclear vacuoles of papillary carcinoma of thyroid observed in fine needle aspiration of thyroid carcinoma. ASCP Check Sample C-80-10 (C-88), 1980.
12. Corwin, T. R.: Medullary carcinoma of the thyroid. *Surg Gynecol Obstet* 138: 453–458, 1974.
13. Soderstrom, N., Telenius-Berg, and Akerman, M.: Diagnosis of medullary carcinoma of the thyroid by fine needle aspiration biopsy. *Acta Med Scand* 197: 71–76, 1975.
14. Ljungberg, O.: Cytologic diagnosis of medullary carcinoma of the thyroid gland with special regard to the demonstration of amyloid in smears of fine needle aspirates. *Acta Cytol* 16(3): 253–255, 1972.
15. Aldinger, K. A., Samaan, N. A., Ibanez, M., and Hill, C. S.: Anaplastic carcinoma of the thyroid: A review of 84 cases of spindle and giant cell carcinoma of the thyroid. *Cancer* 41: 2267–2275, 1978.
16. Persson, P. S.: Cytodiagnosis of thyroiditis. *Acta Med Scand* 183: 1–100, 1967.

The Fluoroscopically Directed
Pulmonary Aspirate

PERSPECTIVES

Aspiration biopsy of the lung is intended for evaluation of the radiographically demonstrable pulmonary lesion. The pragmatic applicability of the procedure complements, if not supersedes conventional fiberoptic bronchoscopy with bronchial brush cytology and cellular examination of sputum. The technique may obviate thoracotomy or contribute information that leads to inclusion of chest surgery in a rational plan of diagnosis, staging, and therapy.

The principal indication is the fundamental necessity to differentiate malignant from benign disease with minimal invasion of the patient and to classify the process reliably so that therapy is accomplished expeditiously. Implicit is the concept of triage in which the cellular composition of the lesion dictates assignment to radiation therapy, chemotherapy, thoracotomy, or surveillance. The cytological diagnosis of small cell undifferentiated carcinoma, oat cell type, obviates thoracotomy and directs referral for radiation or chemotherapy. Squamous cell or adenocarcinoma are conventionally managed with lobectomy or pneumonectomy, and the aspirate confirmation of these patterns complements roentgenographic and clinical evidence for resectability, influencing the decision to operate, or the reticent patient to consent to resection.[1] A judgment of nonresectability may be rescinded when an aspirate diagnosis of malignancy justifies preliminary irradiation that reduces tumor burden,[2] extricating the lesion for excision, or

provides additional data that contradict a premature conclusion from other studies. Dahlgren and Lind[3] reported a case in which bilateral neoplastic involvement was projected by the chest film and the sputum contained undifferentiated carcinoma cells. Aspiration confirmed cancer in one lung, but detected tuberculosis in the other, preserving the patient's candidacy for resection. Nonresectability may be substantiated as an early conclusion by the cytological demonstration of bilateral involvement by a primary lung cancer or confirmation of metastases from an extrapulmonary source. It is particularly advantageous to the cytopathologist if a needle aspirate is available from the primary tumor for comparison with the clinical aspirate. For the patient whose medical restrictions confer a nonresectable status or interdict exploratory thoracotomy, fine needle aspiration cytology provides a method for obtaining tissue-equivalent information.

Aspiration biopsy is somewhat more restricted in analyzing benign lesions because the absence of malignant cells does not unequivocally exclude the possibility of cancer and the cyto-diagnostician must acknowledge this insecurity. Nevertheless, cytopathologists[3,4] have clearly identified benign lesions, such as chondromatous hamartomas, neurofibromas, and bronchial cysts. We have identified a chondromatous hamartoma in one instance, but as yet there has been no surgical confirmation. Sequential radiographic resolution of an indiscretely defined opacification whose cellular sample appeared benign constitutes substantiation of a benign process.

Needle aspiration is effective in acquiring material for the morphological or cultural identification of the causative agents of inflammatory and opportunistic diseases. Dahlgren and Lind[3] correctly detected tuberculosis in six of eight cases in their series when concomitant sputum analysis failed. Johnston and Frable[5] promoted the efficacy of the needle for demonstration of *Pneumocystis carinii,* recommending the Giemsa stain for illustrating the intracystic radial arrangement of the trophozoites. *Candida albicans, Blastomyces dermatitidis,* and *Coccidioides immitis* are readily identified by Papanicolaou's stain, accentuated by periodic acid-Schiff and Gomori's silver methenamine and confirmed by culture. Aerobic and anaerobic cultures may be selected to augment investigation of a lesion that contains fibrinopurulent exudate on the Papanicolaou-stained preparations. The material for special stains or cultures may be obtained by a second pass, or the saline wash of the needle may be used as accessory source material for planting cultures.

The versatility of pulmonary aspiration biopsy is amplified by the accuracy it offers as a diagnostic modality. Pavy[6] reported a rate of 80% and tabulated a range in the literature from 72–87.5%. Zornoza et al.[7] were successful at a rate of 87%. Dahlgren and Nordenstrom,[4] who are credited with provoking recrudescent interest in the technique, have achieved an accuracy of approximately 90%. Dahlgren and Lind[3] in a separate series experienced a rate of 93%, and in a more modest sample Meyer et al.[8] achieved 97%. Despite this facility and accuracy, there has survived an implicit reticence to use the procedure as a primary diagnostic maneuver, and it has been reserved for situations in which bronchoscopy with brushing cytology and sputum analysis have been unrewarding. When the fertility of these alternative procedures was objectively scrutinized, needle aspiration prevailed, providing incentive to investigate with the needle first. Landman et al.[9] compared 100 bronchial brushings and 80 percutaneous needle aspiration biopsies of lung and concluded that although both procedures are valuable and complementary, the diagnostic accuracy of needle biopsy surpasses bronchial brush cytology when the lesions are peripherally located, less than 2.0 cm in diameter, arise in the upper lobes, or do not originate from bronchial epithelium. Dahlgren and Lind[3] compared the needle aspirate sample with concomitant sputum in 125 patients who had at least one satisfactory sputum specimen. Of 101 patients with malignant tumors, 93% were diagnosed by needle aspiration and 64% by sputum cytology. Central origin favors diagnosis by sputum cytology because of access to the bronchial lumina, whereas a peripheral location often precludes exfoliation into the bronchial system and eventual expectoration. The proximity to the periphery confers a high degree of accessibility to the needle probe and promotes aspiration diagnosis of minute and asymptomatic lesions. Sinner[10] reported malignant cells in 106 cases of peripherally situated tumors ranging from 4 mm to 2 cm in diameter. In 80% of the cases, the patients were asymptomatic, surgery was restricted, and perioperative morbidity and mortality were reduced. His conclusions supported aspiration biopsy of the peripheral lesion because early diagnosis resulted in "a better postoperative function of the remaining lung and improved prospects of a final cure." The diagnostic value of aspiration cytology is not dependent on the histological type of the tumor in contradistinction to sputum analysis in which cellular dissociation and exfoliation are a function of the tissue type. All pulmonary carcinomas may be cellular donors to needle acquisition, but small cell undifferentiated carcinomas and adenocarcinomas hesitate to uncouple their cells to dispersion in sputum,[3] whereas squamous and large cell undifferentiated carcinomas are enthusiastic exfoliators. (The peripheral location of the former may explain this phenomenon in part). The procedures are parallel in that increments of sampling predispose to a more lucrative opportunity for a positive diagnosis. The small occult cancer is often more easily diagnosed by sputum cytology in a screening effort, but radiographic visibility is necessary if needle aspiration is to be attempted for investigation of small new primary tumors. Size also influences the efficacy of both techniques in that very large tumors may obstruct a bronchus, inhibiting spontaneous discharge to the exterior for detection, and undergo partial infarction, releasing cellular detritus and inflammatory exudate to the inquisitive needle.

The contraindications to performing fine needle aspiration biopsy of pulmonary lesions have been concisely summarized by Stevens et al.[2] and reiterated by Johnston and Frable.[5] Hemorrhagic diathesis, anticoagulant therapy, and pulmonary hypertension may predispose to intraparenchymal hemorrhage or hemoptysis following insertion of the needle and readjustment during the evacuation maneuver. Uncontrolled cough may deflect the needle from target, inflicting trauma to delicate parenchymal or more substantial vasculature. Arteriovenous malformations as reservoirs of blood threaten extravasation from the puncture wounds. Advanced emphysema complicated by bullae inflicts pneumothorax as a complication that may require insertion of a chest tube for reinflation. Puncture of an hydatid cyst should be avoided to prevent dispersion of scoleces throughout the thoracic cavity. If these contraindications are observed and case selection is rational, serious complications may be averted.

Complications that have been described, if not overdramatized, have included pneumothorax, bleeding, air embolism, and implantation of tumor cells along the needle tract.

Stevens et al.[2] reported pneumothorax in 39 instances following 126 procedures (31%): most were small, asymptomatic, and resolved spontaneously, but nine required placement of a chest tube because of dyspnea. This experience is representative of most reports concerning pneumothorax and further contributes the postulate that the occurrence of pneumothorax may be a function of the frequency of passes. Pneumothorax was the only significant complication in the series of Fontana et al.[1] affecting about half the patients and requiring intrapleural suction in about a third of these. In 16 of Sinner's[10] 163 needle biopsies a small pneumothorax was observed with a 1–2 cm rim of apical air that was spontaneously resorbed; nine additional patients had a more substantial pneumothorax requiring

suction of air, but in only one patient was there sufficient clinical compromise to require a chest tube. Dahlgren and Lind[3] referred to "pneumothorax of some degree," particularly in patients with emphysema, but did not emphasize this as a serious complication in their mammoth series of more than 3000 aspirates. The implication is strong that pneumothorax is routinely encountered and should not dissuade the medical community from implementing aspiration biopsy of the lung. Zornoza et al.[7] indicated that his rate of pneumothorax declined with experience: an over-all rate of 14% was contrasted with 6% in his last 50 cases.

Hemorrhage after aspiration did not occur in the Scandinavian experience[3] or in Zornoza et al.'s[7] series. Fontana et al.[1] reported six insignificant episodes of hemoptysis. In Sinner's[10] series from Stockholm, local bleeding from the puncture site occurred in 14 of the 163 aspirates, but was spontaneously resorbed; there was no hemoptysis recorded. Stevens et al.[2] described brief hemoptysis in the form of blood-tinged sputum and bleeding stopped within minutes. One small hemopneumothorax was apparently clinically insignificant. Milner et al.[11] reported the fifth fatality in the literature following aspiration biopsy of the lung. The patient exsanguinated from trauma to a muscular artery, despite his meticulous selection for the procedure after exclusion of the contraindications. Zelch and Lalli[12] provided reassurance from their series of more than 700 aspirations that bleeding is not a major complication, despite entry of the needle into the thoracic aorta, right atrium, pulmonary arteries and veins, and the vena cava without

TABLE I
Pulmonary Aspirates with Surgical Follow-up

Cytology	Tissue	Number
Positive	Positive	41
Positive	Negative	4
Suspicious	Negative	1
Negative	Positive	2
Negative	Negative	15
Negative	Unsatisfactory	2
Unsatisfactory	Unsatisfactory	1
Total		66

untoward effects. In one instance in our personal experience we inadvertently entered the aortic arch in an attempt to sample an adjacent squamous cell carcinoma. The puncture wound sealed spontaneously and there was no bleeding.

Air embolism is clinically insignificant because of the small diameter of the needle.

Translocation of tumor cells to the needle tract with contamination of contiguous structures is an irrational fear based on rare anecdotal evidence. Two occurrences in Dahlgren and Lind's series[3] of 3000 aspirates were related to highly malignant, aggressive undifferentiated cancers that would predictably disseminate with spontaneity. Pavy et al.[6] quoted Wolinsky's account of needle tract implantation, but the larger-core Franklin-Silverman needle was the offending implement. The other major series annotated in the discussion of complications did not experience needle tract dissemination of tumor as a sequel of concern.

Our experience with fluoroscopically directed fine needle aspiration cytology at the Eisenhower Medical Center encompassed a 3-year period from 1978 through 1980 and included 130 cases. Fifty-three patients were females, ages 25–90 years, and 77 were males, ages 27–83 years. The size of the aspirated lesions varied in diameter from 0.8–12.0 cm. Biopsy or autopsy tissue confirmation was available for 66 cases, and relationship of cytological projection to tissue diagnosis is summarized in Table I. Forty-five malignancies were diagnosed cytologically and substantiated by biopsy in 41 cases. The four cases in which biopsy was noncorrelative provided unequivocal radiographic or clinical evidence for malignancy, but the bronchoscopic biopsy forceps failed to reach the tumor, or a benign supraclavicular lymph node was sampled. Our accuracy rate in this limited series therefore exceeds the statistics of Nordenstrom and Dahlgren.[4] The positive tissue analyses included 19 resections (lobectomy or pneumonectomy), five lymph node biopsies, one bone marrow biopsy, six lung biopsies, nine resections of primary lesions responsible for the metastatic envoys, and one autopsy. Of the 19 resections, the lesion resided in the left upper lobe in four instances, in the right upper lobe in 11, right lower lobe in two, and left lower lobe in two. In the overwhelming majority of cases, the cell-type projected by the aspirate was confirmed by the histopathology; one discrepancy was in the cytological interpretation of a small round cell lesion as probable lymphoma; the tissue proved to represent oat cell carcinoma. The records are incomplete with respect to the occurrence of pneumothorax. Of a sample of 56 charts

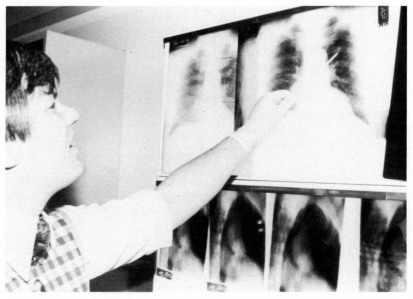

Fig. 5-1. Dr. Richard Lynch, radiologist, localizes the pulmonary lesion on the chest roentgenogram.

inspected, there were 26 reports of pneumothorax (46% incidence), but only seven required the placement of chest tubes for pulmonary reinflation and the patients were not compromised. Three of the 26 developed transient subcutaneous emphysema. There was no serious hemorrhage, although occasional patients would produce a singular expectorate of blood-tinged mucus. Neither air embolism nor transfer implantation of malignant cells along the needle path are known to have occurred.

Technical Suggestions

The procedure we utilize is a modification of the technique of Dahlgren and Nordenstrom[4] and is dependent on image-intensified fluoroscopic placement of a 22-gauge flexible spinal needle (with stylet) in the lesion. We do not have the advantage of biplane fluoroscopy or a C-arm for two-dimensional perspectives and must therefore estimate the depth of the lesion and the optimal angle for penetration. The patient is placed horizontally within the cardiac cradle of the fluoroscopy table in a position that is advantageous to approach the lesion. The cytopathologist and cytotechnologist assistant are notified and the attending radiologist reviews the pertinent chest roentgenograms with them prior to initiating the procedure (Fig. 5-1). The skin is prepared with a disinfectant solution and is anesthetized with 1% Xylocaine, which is allowed to penetrate the deeper tissues. The lesion is local-

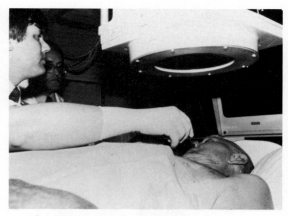

Fig. 5-3. Readjustment of the thin needle.

ized fluoroscopically and the needle is inserted to a depth estimated by comparing actual lateral chest measurements with the knowledge of the relative magnification of the lateral chest film as described by Stevens et al.[2] (Fig. 5-2). The needle is readjusted (Figs. 5-3, 5-4) until there is a unison of motion of needle tip and the lesion during respiratory excursions. Rotation of the patient in the cardiac cradle may facilitate assessment of needle position on the television monitor (Figs. 5-5–5-7). Johnson and Frable[5] used paper clips and tape to localize small lesions, depending on the skin imprint of the

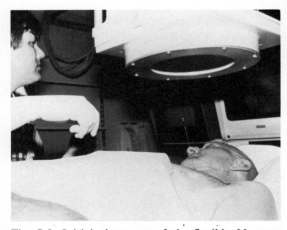

Fig. 5-2. Initial placement of the flexible 22-gauge spinal needle for fluoroscopic localization of the lesion.

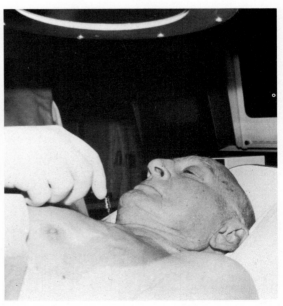

Fig. 5-4. Deep insertion of the needle with stylet in place.

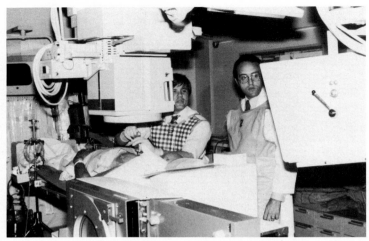

Fig. 5-5. Radiologist and pathologist consult the television monitor for the position of the needle with respect to the lesion.

paperclip for the needle entry site. Stevens et al.[2] found it helpful to obtain tomograms while the patient is in the biopsy position. "By Caliper measurement of the tabletop-needle entry site distance and subtraction of the tomographically determined tabletop-lesion distance, one can determine the approximate lesion depth from the skin surface." When the needle tip reaches its appropriate destination (Fig. 5-8), the stylet is removed and a disposable 20-cc syringe without Luer lock is attached (Fig. 5-9). The plunger is withdrawn to create a vacuum and the needle is

repositioned in various planes (Figs. 5-10, 5-11). The needle is withdrawn only after the vacuum has been allowed to re-equilibrate in order to avoid displacement of the material from the lumen of the needle into the barrel of the syringe (Fig. 5-12). The needle and syringe are immediately given to the cytopathologist (Fig. 5-13) who removes the needle to reintroduce air into the syringe (Fig. 5-14). This provides an expulsive force to displace the aspirated material from the core of the needle to glass slides (Fig. 5-15). Droplets are released at the end of the slides opposite the frosted labels and the slides are placed in contact to permit dispersion of the liquid material in a circular monolayer, concentrating the screening field to one locale (Fig. 5-16). The slides are separated in a perpendicular direction to avoid smearing the material and are immediately immersed in 95% ethanol for fixation (Fig. 5-17). A minimum of 3 minutes is allowed for fixation and the slides are stained by a rapid variant of the Papanicolaou's technique (Fig. 5-18), while the patient is retained in position on the fluoroscopy table. A rapid analysis is provided, the quality of the material is assessed, and a diagnosis is rendered if possible. If material is inadequate or an additional specimen is required for special stains or culture, a second pass is conveniently done. The needle is rinsed in physiological saline to provide a liquid medium from which cultures or cell membrane preparations can be done. Immediate and 2-hour

Fig. 5-6. The television monitor aides in the appropriate guidance of the needle to its destination.

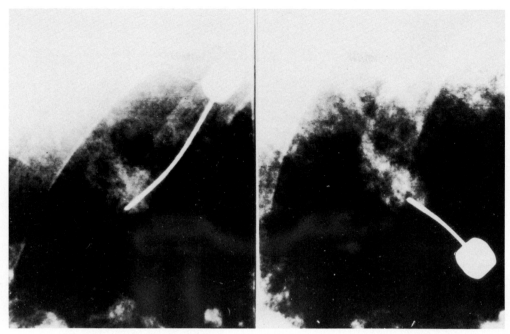

Fig. 5-7. Radiographic demonstration of the needle in situ within the lesion.

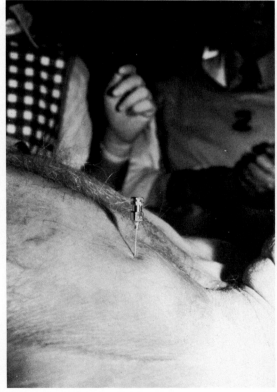

Fig. 5-8. The needle is in place and the stylet can be exchanged for the syringe.

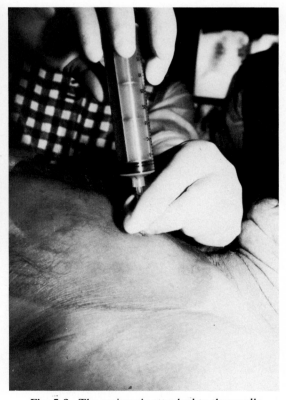

Fig. 5-9. The syringe is attached to the needle.

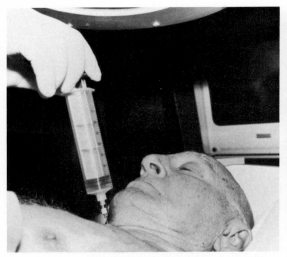

Fig. 5-10. The radiologist withdraws the plunger to create a vacuum in the syringe.

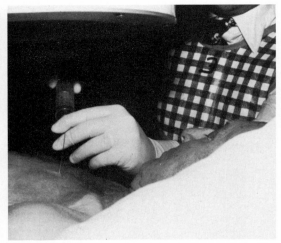

Fig. 5-12. The needle is withdrawn.

postbiopsy chest films are taken for assessment of complications, such as pneumothorax, and may be repeated at 24 hours if indicated. All patients are hospitalized for the procedure and postbiopsy surveillance. We insist on the availability of the cytopathologist or cytotechnologist for acquisition and processing of the material to achieve optimal diagnosis and clinical correlation.

CELLS FROM PARENCHYMAL NODULES

The pulmonary harvest is a collage of fascinating cellular images whose intricacies of shape, nuclear texture, and cytoplasmic posture intertwine to project a portrait of tissue systems,

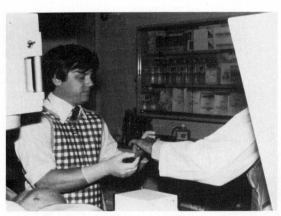

Fig. 5-13. Needle and syringe are given to the pathologist.

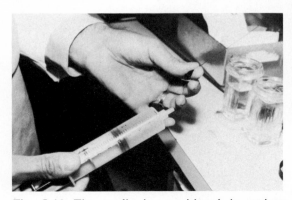

Fig. 5-11. The needle is repositioned in various planes.

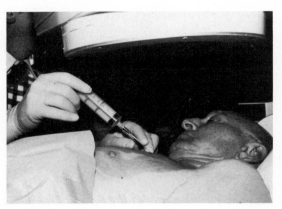

Fig. 5-14. The pathologist disconnects the needle from the syringe to introduce air for an expulsive force.

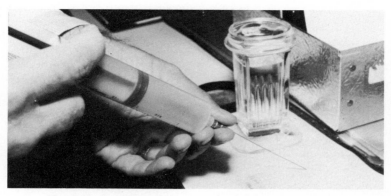

Fig. 5-15. Aspirated material is expressed onto glass slides.

awarding identity to a neoplasm or inflammatory process. There is an inherent artform to be applauded that surpasses an impressionist's perspective and focuses on the detail of a cellular tapestry, 10 or 12 elements in a mosaic that reflect the total form and structure of a more comprehensive phenomenon requiring accent, definition. Needle aspiration of the lung provides a versatile and creative approach to pulmonary diagnosis within this perspective.

Through a series of brief encounters with patients whose pulmonary infiltrates or opacities were analyzed by needle aspiration cytology, we hope to communicate the spectrum of disease that can be defined by aspiration biopsy and illustrate the appearance in the medium of aspiration cytology of common and unusual, neoplastic and inflammatory abberrations that affect the lungs.

A 69-year-old male with antecedent history of chronic obstructive pulmonary disease and rheumatoid arthritis treated with corticosteroids was admitted for evaluation of hemoptysis and pulmonary distress. Chest roentgenograms

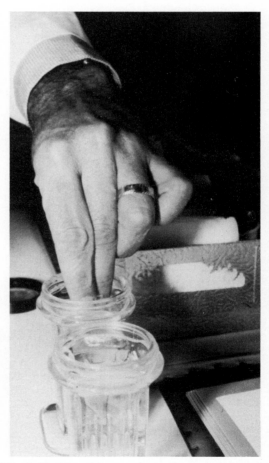

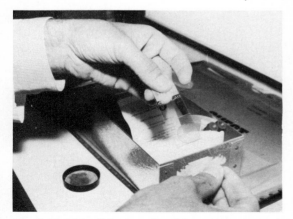

Fig. 5-16. Two slides are placed in contact to permit monolayer dispersion of the cellular aspirate.

Fig. 5-17. The slides are immediately immersed in ethanol for rapid fixation.

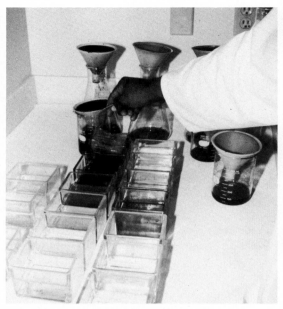

Fig. 5-18. The slides are stained by a rapid variant of Papanicolaou's technique.

(Figs. 5-19, 5-20) demonstrated a cavitary mass in the right upper lobe. Fine needle aspiration preparations (Figs. 5-21, 5-22) demonstrated tenuously cohesive cells with nuclei exhibiting

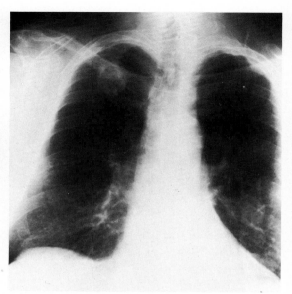

Fig. 5-20. Chest x-ray, anteroposterior (AP) projection demonstrating lesion in right upper lobe.

considerable anisokaryosis, homogenization of chromatin, angularity, fusiform tapering of peripheral contours, and irregular convolutional serration of envelopes. Cytoplasm varied in quantity, but generally presented a quality of hyaline homogenization. Individually dissociated elements appeared overtly keratinized (Fig. 5-22). Fragments of cytoplasm and nuclear remnants constituted a diathesis.

A lobectomy was performed on the basis of the aspirate diagnosis and the resected tumor measured approximately 4 cm in diameter and presented a peripheral rim of gray-white, lobulated, homogeneous friable tissue circumscribing a central cavity with hemorrhagic debris (Fig. 5-23). Microscopic sections confirmed the cytological diagnosis of invasive squamous cell carcinoma. In many areas, the tissue reflected a microcosm of the gross lesion with a peripheral lobulated zone of viable cellularity surrounding a central area of acantholysis with degenerating keratinized cells dissociated from parent aggregates. The cellular constituents were arranged in tight mosaics (Fig. 5-24) with a tendency to form epithelial pearls (Fig. 5-25). Nuclei exhibited changes of vesicularity, coarse chromatin dispersion, and irregularities of contour, but the extreme hyperchromasia and homogenization seen in the Papanicolaou-stained material was

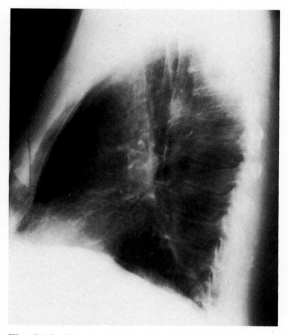

Fig. 5-19. Chest x-ray demonstrating lateral view of lesion in right upper lobe.

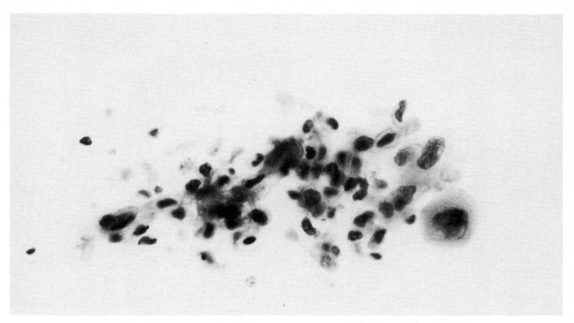

Fig. 5-21. Needle aspirate, Papanicolaou's stain, 625×, squamous cell carcinoma.

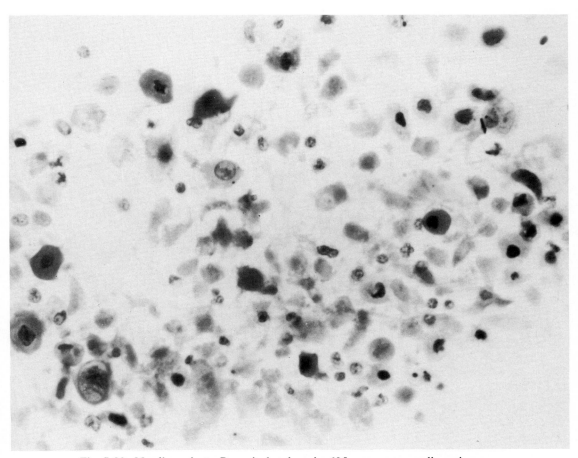

Fig. 5-22. Needle aspirate, Papanicolaou's stain, 625×, squamous cell carcinoma.

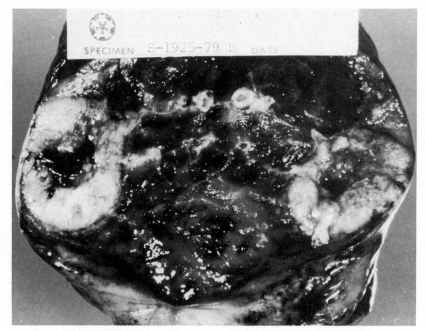

Fig. 5-23. Lobectomy specimen with cavitary squamous cell carcinoma.

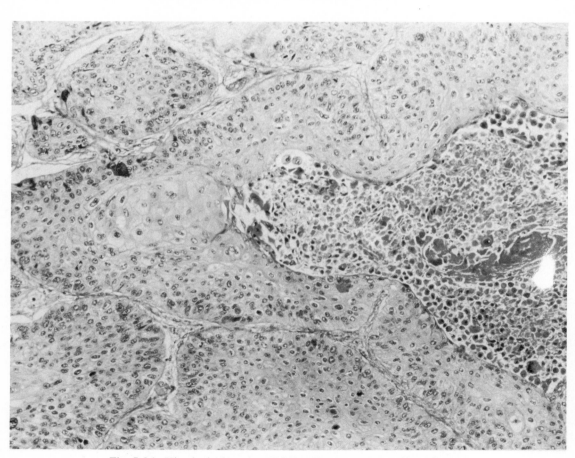

Fig. 5-24. Histological section, H&E, 160×, squamous cell carcinoma.

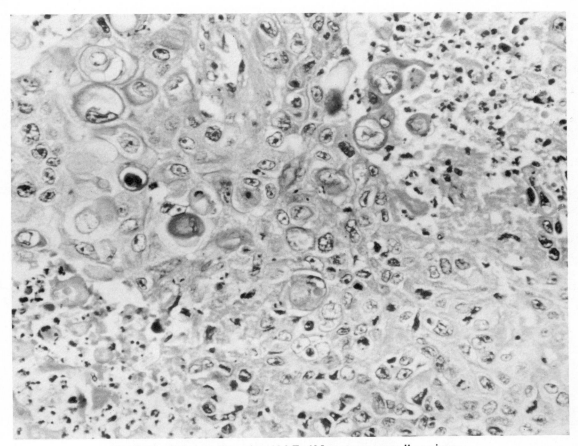

Fig. 5-25. Histological section, H&E, 625×, squamous cell carcinoma.

not transferred to the tissue, except in areas of central acantholysis and keratinization. The cytomorphological features illustrated by this case are characteristic of our experience with squamous cell carcinoma investigated by this technique, although some lesions may exhibit more of a tendency to spindling of cells with large, anaplastic variants included in the cellular population. The patient died on the 19th postoperative day from *Pseudomonas* pneumonitis and progressive pulmonary insufficiency. Autopsy was denied.

A 67-year-old male smoker was evaluated for complaint of chest pain, back pain, and weight loss. A chest x-ray demonstrated a 3 cm mass in the left upper lobe associated with left hilar adenopathy (Fig. 5-26). Bronchoscopy and mediastinoscopy were negative and the patient was referred for thin needle aspiration of the left upper lobe mass and hilar lesion. The peripheral

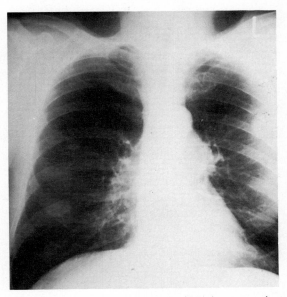

Fig. 5-26. Chest x-ray, AP projection demonstrating mass in left upper lobe.

aspirate contained necrotic tissue without definitive tumor cells. The hilar aspiration biopsy (Figs. 5-27, 5-28) provided a highly cellular sample, which illustrates the cytological characteristics of adenocarcinoma in this medium. The individual cells are arranged in sheets, cords, and acinar configurations. Although cytoplasm is abundant and granular or delicately vacuolated, margins are indistinct and there is suggestion of syncytial confluence. Nuclear contour is subtly variable with occasional indentations or projections, but the envelopes are crisply delimited. The nucleoplasm is vesicular with punctately stippled, regular chromatin granules and aggregates. Nucleoli are prominent, smoothly circumscribed, slightly eccentric, and dominate the nuclear structure. Mucicarmine stains provided confirmatory evidence to substantiate glandular origin or differentiation. A postbiopsy film (Fig.

5-29) demonstrated a persistent, asymptomatic 20–30% pneumothorax that was expected to resolve spontaneously. Because of a positive bone scan accounting for the clinical back pain, the patient was considered inoperable and was referred to a medical oncologist.

This case illustrates several important concepts: needle aspiration is the procedure of choice for establishing a cytological diagnosis of malignancy and could have been elected as a primary procedure rather than an alternate to unsuccessful bronchoscopy and mediastinoscopy; pneumothorax is to be anticipated with multiple passes, occurs without clinically significant embarassment, and can often be expected to resolve without further intervention; aspiration biopsy can obviate thoracotomy in establishing a specific diagnosis of cancer, including cell type, and establish the nonresectability or inoperabil-

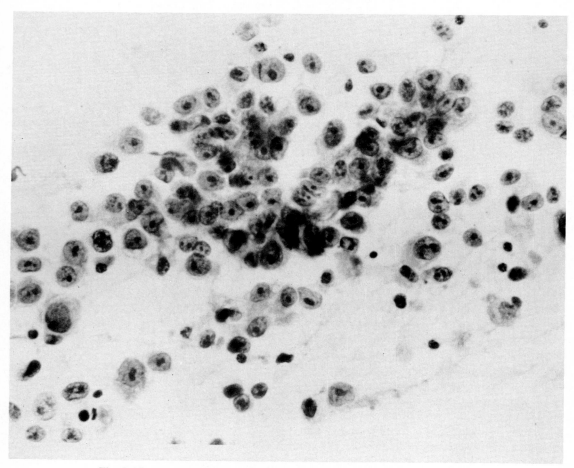

Fig. 5-27. Needle aspirate, Papanicolaou's stain, 500×, adenocarcinoma.

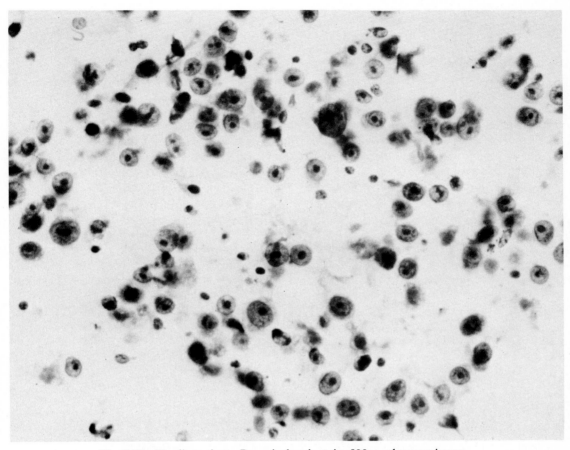

Fig. 5-28. Needle aspirate, Papanicolaou's stain, 500×, adenocarcinoma.

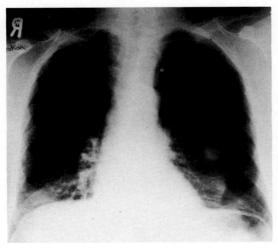

Fig. 5-29. Postbiopsy chest x-ray, AP projection demonstrating 20–30% pneumothorax.

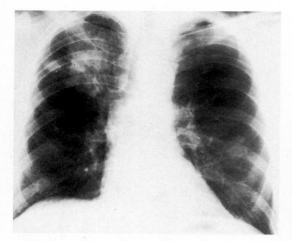

Fig. 5-30. Chest x-ray, AP projection demonstrating mass in right upper lobe.

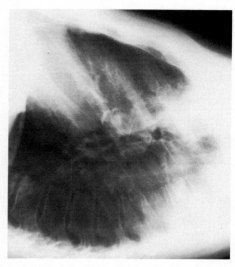

Fig. 5-31. Chest x-ray, lateral projection demonstrating mass in left upper lobe.

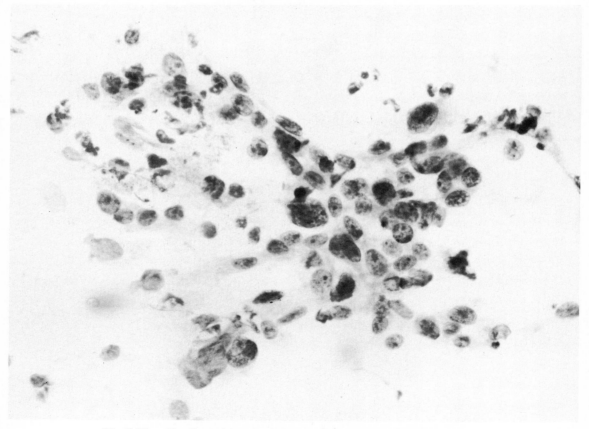

Fig. 5-32 a. Needle aspirate, Papanicolaou's stain, 400×, adenocarcinoma.

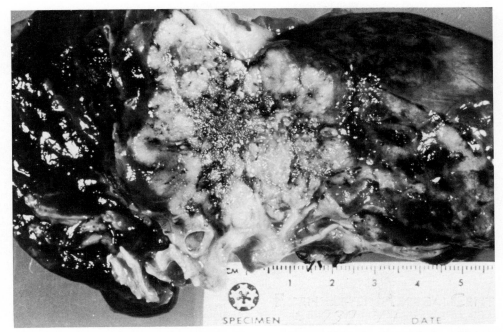

Fig. 5-32 b. Lobectomy specimen demonstrating apical segmental bronchus in contiguity with tumor.

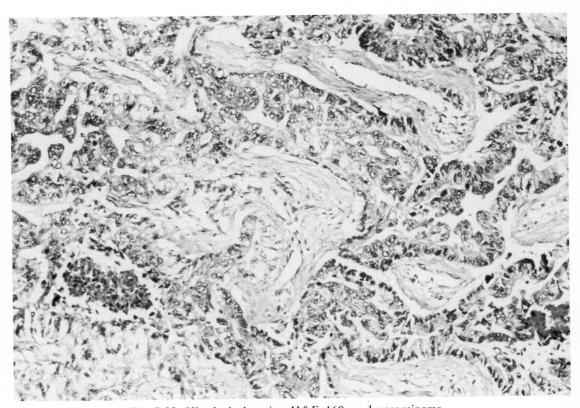

Fig. 5-33. Histological section, H&E, 160×, adenocarcinoma.

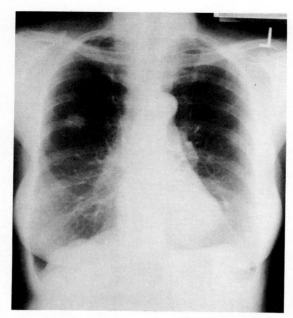

Fig. 5-34. Chest film, AP projection demonstrating lesion in right upper lobe.

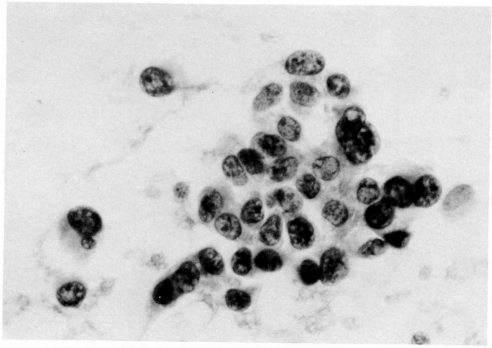

Fig. 5-35. Needle aspirate, Papanicolaou's stain, 625×, adenocarcinoma.

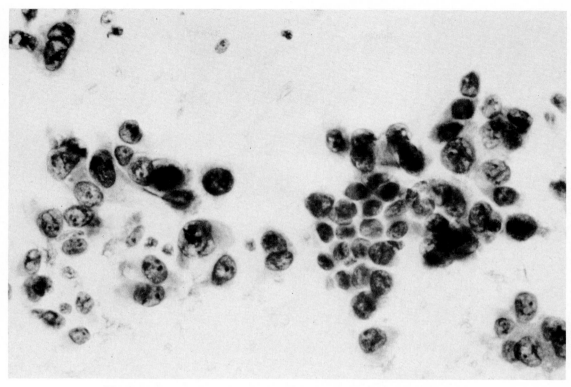

Fig. 5-36. Needle aspirate, Papanicolaou's stain, 500×, adenocarcinoma.

ity status of the patient who hosts disseminated cancer. Expeditious referral to the medical oncologist or radiotherapist is then mandated.

Poorly differentiated adenocarcinoma is exemplified by an aspirate from a 60-year-old male with a large opacity in the right upper lobe extending to pleura (Figs. 5-30, 5-31). The luxuriant aspirate contained cells loosely aggregated within sunburst arrangements. Although abortive acinar formations are invoked, a definitive glandular pattern is not respected. The nuclei vary in size, shape, and chromatinic quality, with variable stages of preservation or deterioration. The granular cytoplasm is communal with indistinct borders (Fig. 5-32 a). A right upper lobectomy was accomplished on the basis of the aspirate report. The apical segmental bronchus was contiguous with a granular, gray-white neoplasm measuring 5 by 5 by 2.5 cm in direct contiguity with pleura (Fig. 5-32 b).

Histological sections confirmed poorly differentiated cells arranged in sheets with a vaguely arborescent and pseudopapillary character (Fig. 5-33). This appearance is repeated in the cytological assessment of a 72-year-old woman with a small coin lesion in the right upper lobe (Fig. 5-34). Well-preserved glandular cells with columnar silhouettes are related around a central space that corresponds to a luminal crevice (Fig. 5-35). The cytoplasm is well defined, granular, or vacuolated, with visible boundaries. Nucleoli are not particularly prominent, camouflaged in some cells by the coarsely stippled chromatinic environment. Other fields demonstrate considerably more aberration in nuclear sizes and shapes (Fig. 5-36). The lobectomy specimen provided histological confirmation of serrated glandular units composing the neoplasm (Fig. 5-37). A right middle lobe mass in a 43-year-old male smoker (Figs. 5-38, 5-39) was evaluated by aspiration biopsy and the hyperchromatic, monomorphic cell population was organized into acinar structures. This configuration was the clue that permitted appropriate categorization as an adenocarcinoma (Fig. 5-40), because other fields in which the

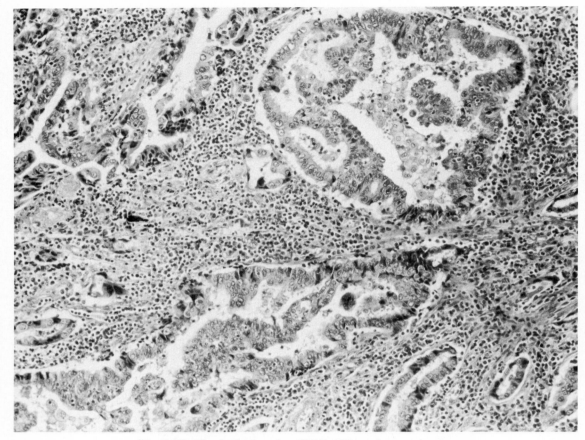

Fig. 5-37. Histological section, H&E, 160×, adenocarcinoma.

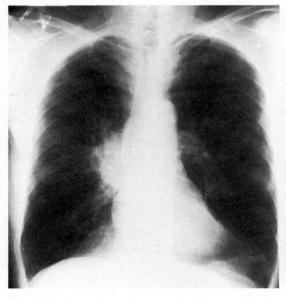

Fig. 5-38. Chest film, AP projection demonstrating a right middle lobe mass.

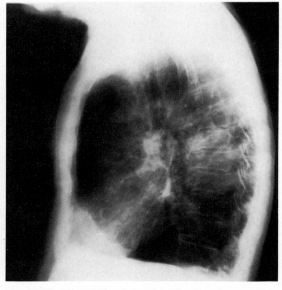

Fig. 5-39. Chest film, lateral projection demonstrating right middle lobe mass.

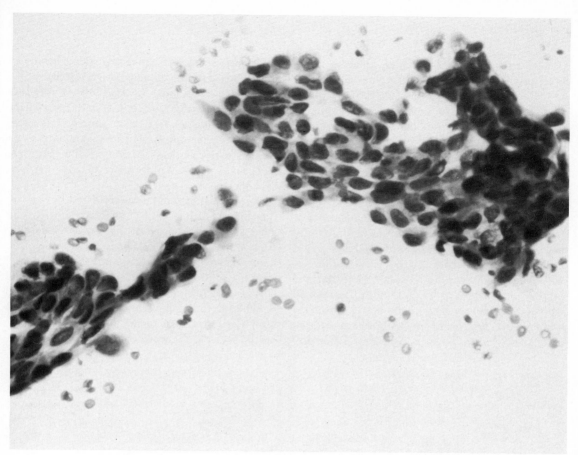

Fig. 5-40. Needle aspirate, Papanicolaou's stain, 400×, adenocarcinoma.

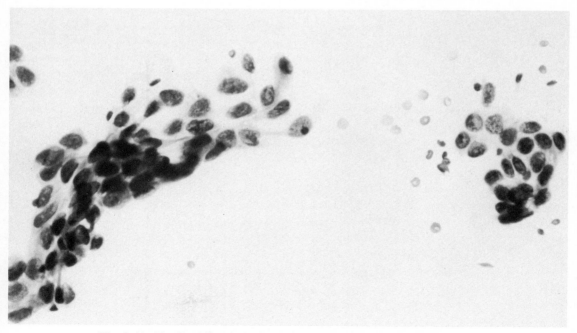

Fig. 5-41. Needle aspirate, Papanicolaou's stain, 400×, adenocarcinoma.

143

pattern was lacking (Fig. 5-41) could be interpreted only as anaplastic carcinoma. The corresponding tissue preparations disclosed organization into acini with intraluminal papillary upheaval (Fig. 5-42) and bizarre nuclear anaplasia (Fig. 5-43). A final example of primary adenocarcinoma of lung observed as a routine preparation is the aspirate from a 53-year-old woman with a left upper lobe mass (Fig. 5-44) and a glandular pattern (Fig. 5-45).

Our experience with bronchioloalveolar carcinoma has been infrequent, and the aspirate diagnosis, if isolated from the clinical history and radiographic appearance, may be quite difficult. The roentgenographic display of bilateral billowy opacifications (Fig. 5-46 a) combined with a cellular appearance of bland, vesicular nuclei with prominent nucleoli in vacuolated cytoplasm that projects a columnar silhouette

constitute strong evidence for this variant of pulmonary adenocarcinoma (Fig. 5-46 b).

Primary carcinoma of the lung is often a composite of histoarchitectural patterns and the probing needle may select a sample that accurately reflects the constituent population, or inadvertently neglects a component. Multiple passes may secure a more representative analytical cohort.

A 61-year-old female was referred for aspiration biopsy of a poorly defined solitary 1.5 cm mass in the left upper lobe that progressed under surveillance (Fig. 5-47). The lesion was localized fluoroscopically with image-intensification and impaled with a flexible 22-gauge spinal needle (Fig. 5-48). A biphasic cellular population could be discriminated. Several clusters of large cells with hyperchromatic nuclei and prominent chromatin precipitates were conjugated by intercel-

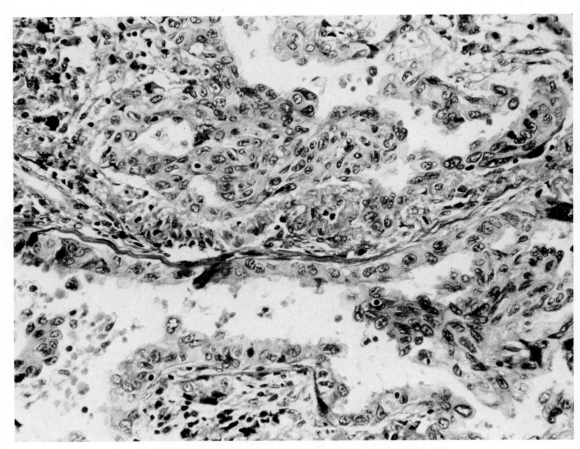

Fig. 5-42. Histological section, H&E, 315×, adenocarcinoma.

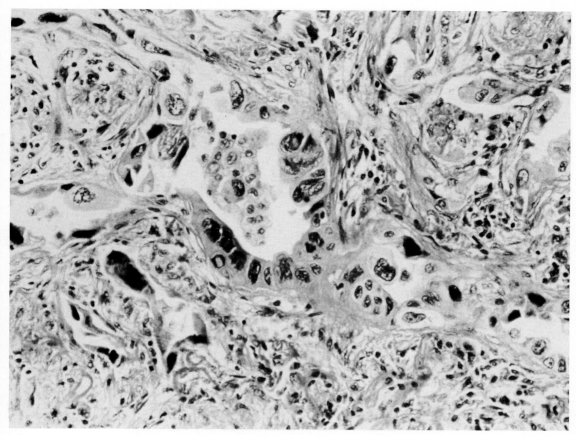

Fig. 5-43. Histological section, H&E, 315×, adenocarcinoma.

Fig. 5-44. Chest film, AP projection demonstrating left upper lobe mass.

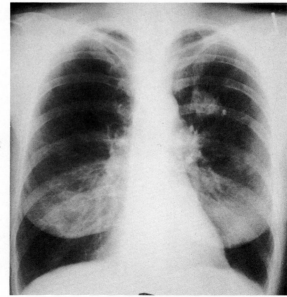

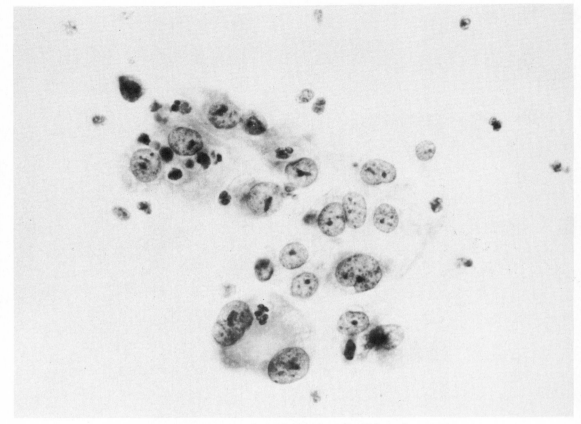

Fig. 5-45. Needle aspirate, Papanicolaou's stain, 625×, adenocarcinoma.

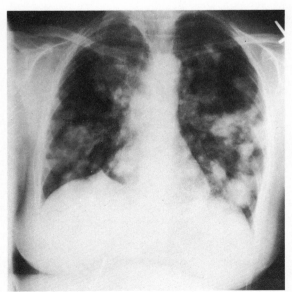

Fig. 5-46 a. Chest film, AP projection demonstrating nodular, bilateral billowy infiltrates.

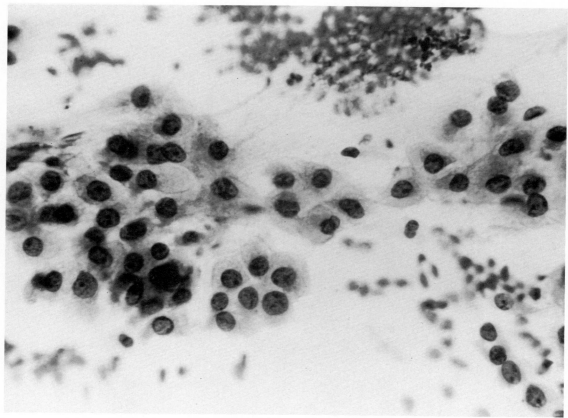

Fig. 5-46 b. Needle aspirate, Papanicolaou's stain, 400×, bronchiolar variant of adenocarcinoma.

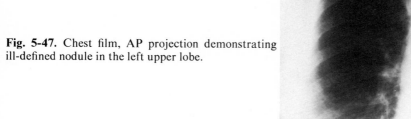

Fig. 5-47. Chest film, AP projection demonstrating ill-defined nodule in the left upper lobe.

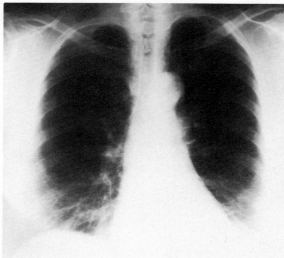

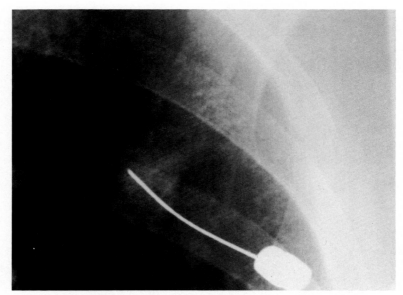

Fig. 5-48. Intensified fluoroscopic image of lesion impaled on needle.

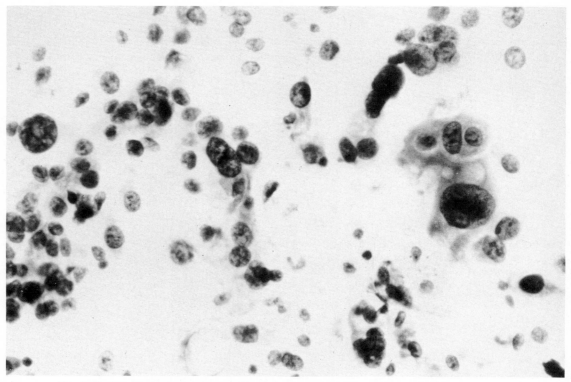

Fig. 5-49. Needle aspirate, Papanicolaou's stain, 500×, mixed adenosquamous carcinoma.

lular cytoplasmic filaments, implicating derivation from a squamous orientation (Fig. 5-49). Isolated, dissociated fusiform cells were arbitrarily dispersed (Fig. 5-50). Adjacent aggregates of small cells with indeterminate cytoplasmic boundaries and nondescript nuclei with coarse hyperchromasia formed arbitrary nests and trabecular cords, and glandular features were invoked on a visceral, if not scientific, basis. The lesion was resected by restricted lobectomy and presented as a subpleural 1.8 cm sphere (Fig. 5-51).

Microscopically, intimate comingling of squamoid cells in a tight mosaic with mucicarmine-positive, small cuboidal cells often arranged with intraluminal pseudopapillary upheaval, provided substantive evidence for a mixed carcinoma (Fig. 5-52 a & b). In this instance, the aspiration biopsy accurately predicted structure of the small tumor. The patient was released to clinical surveillance without additional therapy.

A 32-year-old woman who worked as a chemical engineer was evaluated for cough secondary to a mass involving the right middle and lower lobes (Figs. 5-53, 5-54). A fluoroscopically directed needle aspirate retrieved anaplastic cells arbitrarily arranged in cohesive clusters (Fig. 5-55). The nuclei appeared definitively malignant, but there were no specific patterns of relationship to suggest a glandular or squamoid preference. A contiguous right middle and lower lobectomy were performed and the tumor consisted of a solid, homogeneous, gray-white neoplasm measuring 7.5 by 6.0 by 5.0 cm contained within a trabeculated, deflated cyst (Fig. 5-56). The histological sections confirmed sheets of anaplastic cells of intermediate size in an amorphous composite (Fig. 5-57), corroborat-

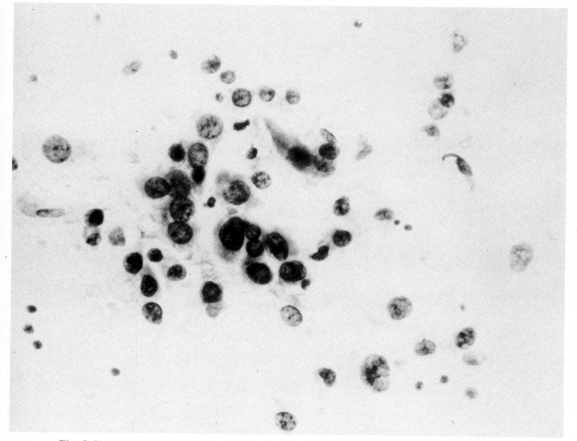

Fig. 5-50. Needle aspirate, Papanicolaou's stain, 500×, mixed adenosquamous carcinoma.

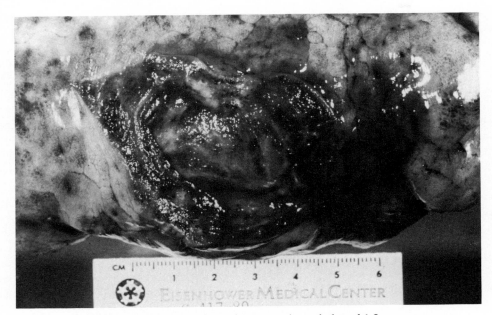

Fig. 5-51. Lobectomy specimen demonstrating subpleural 1.8 cm mass.

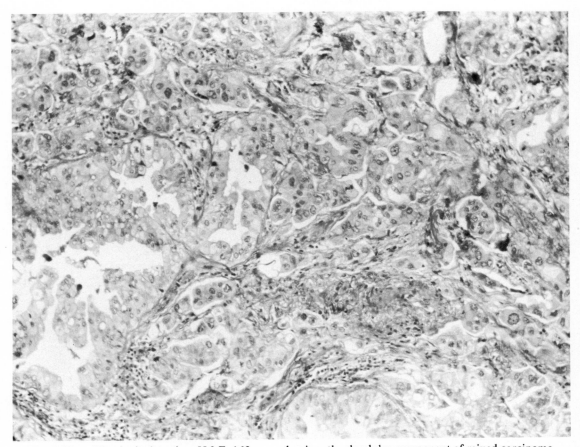

Fig. 5-52 a. Histological section, H&E, 160×, predominantly glandular component of mixed carcinoma.

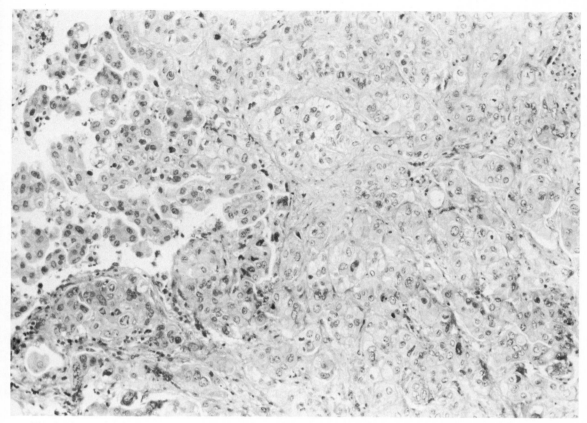

Fig. 5-52 b. Histological section, H&E, 160×, predominantly squamoid component of mixed carcinoma.

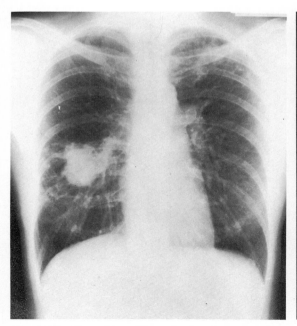

Fig. 5-53. Chest film, AP projection demonstrating mass in right upper and middle lobes.

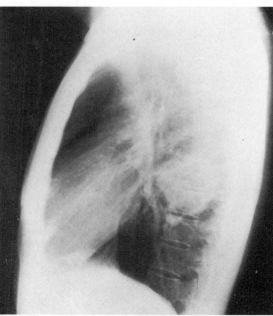

Fig. 5-54. Chest film, lateral projection accentuating mass in right lung.

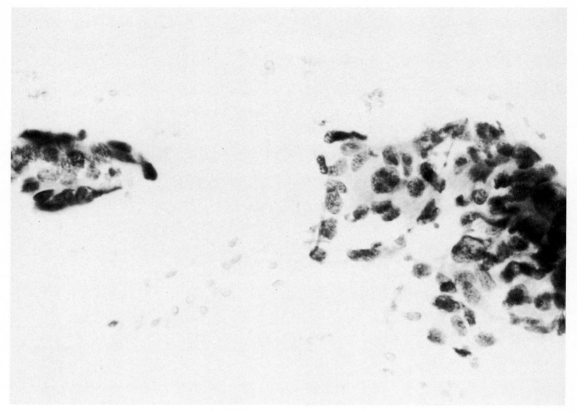

Fig. 5-55. Needle aspirate, Papanicolaou's stain, 500×, anaplastic carcinoma.

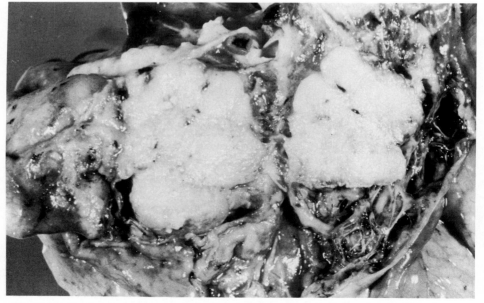

Fig. 5-56. Partial pneumonectomy specimen with neoplasm in deflated trabeculated cyst.

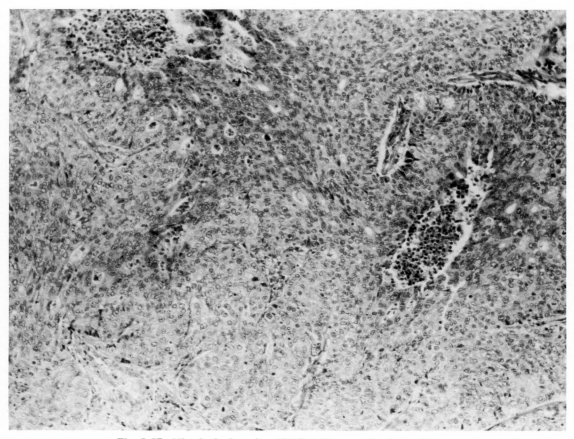

Fig. 5-57. Histological section, H&E, 160×, anaplastic carcinoma.

ing the cytological impressions, but contributed an alternate pattern of glandular units juxtaposed to form a cribriform network of columnar cells with mucus-positive cytoplasmic vacuoles and intraluminal papillary projections (Fig. 5-58). This component was never detected by the aspiration procedure. This is a limitation of consequence when needle aspiration is the sole diagnostic maneuver because the formulation of the chemotherapeutic regimen relies heavily on selection of drug combinations to attack specific structural entities. The full therapeutic benefit may be indirectly and inadvertently denied the patient. In this case, the anaplastic component was the critical element clinically:tumor metastasized abruptly to the face, a bronchopleural fistula developed, empyema supervened, and the patient succumbed to her tumor, which progressed with vicious and almost deliberate peregrinations. Sampling omissions can be reduced, but not eliminated if there are multiple passes directed at various positions within the localized lesion, avoiding the necrotic center, and if the pathologist is insistent on adequate cellularity before validating the specimen as appropriate for interpretative assay.

Sinner and Sandstedt[13] have reiterated the British Medical Research Council's reinforcement of the opinion that small cell undifferentiated carcinoma, oat cell type, may be an absolute contraindication to operation, and that radiation or chemotherapy are the preferred alternatives. The inordinate value of fine needle aspiration cytology as an atraumatic method of acquiring cells to substantiate this diagnosis and obviate thoracotomy is virtually self-evident. In the series reported previously, small cell anaplastic carcinoma was diagnosed cytologically in 54 of 2726 consecutive transthoracic fine needle aspiration biopsies and found to be a reliable

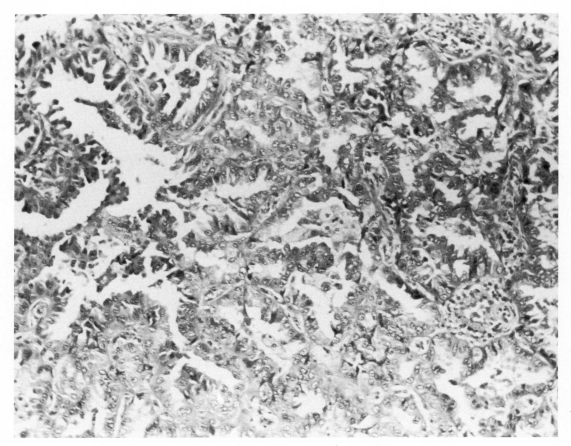

Fig. 5-58. Histological section, H&E, 160×, adenocarcinoma component.

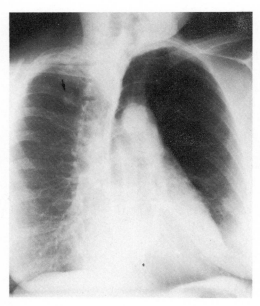

Fig. 5-59. Chest film, AP projection demonstrating small peripheral lesion in right upper lobe.

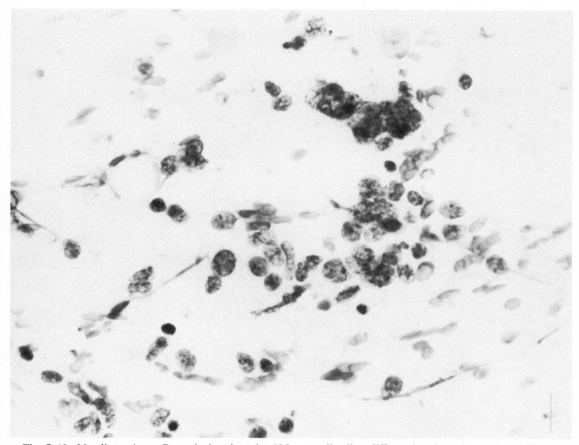

Fig. 5-60. Needle aspirate, Papanicolaou's stain, 625×, small cell undifferentiated carcinoma, oat cell type.

diagnostic method in correlation with clinical findings and roentgenograms. This opinion was based on histological evidence available in 31 instances with corroboration of oat cell carcinoma in 28 cases.

Three illustrative cases demonstrate the diagnosis and confirmation of undifferentiated carcinoma, small cell (oat cell) and intermediate cell types. In these instances, surgical intervention was elected and provided tissue for correlative comparisons. A 1 cm nodule was detected by routine chest x-ray in the right upper lobe of an asymptomatic 67-year-old woman (Fig. 5-59) and was subjected to aspiration biopsy under fluoroscopic guidance. The cellular population was immediately characterized as a small cell undifferentiated lesion (Figs. 5-60, 5-61) on the basis of size parameters, minimal cytoplasm, and round or fusiform nuclei in juxtaposition with molding, coarse chromatin dispersion, and

absent nucleoli. Intimate contact of six or eight cells in unified clusters was contradicted by dissociated single elements. The nuclear patterns were reminiscent of activated lymphocytes but communal tendency and spindling, the deteriorated quality of some elements and the indentations in nuclear envelopes imposed by affiliate neighbors imposed an epithelial aura.

Because of the small size of the parent lesion, its peripheral location and fortuitous discovery, negative radionuclide survey, bronchoscopy, mediastinoscopy, and bone marrow examination, it was elected to perform a lobectomy. The tumor was a 1 cm, circumscribed, homogeneous, gray-white nodule insinuated beneath the pleura (Fig. 5-62). Histological preparations at two levels of magnification (Figs. 5-63, 5-64) confirmed the development of an undifferentiated carcinoma beneath the intact epithelial layer of the segmental bronchus. The cells were disported in sheets,

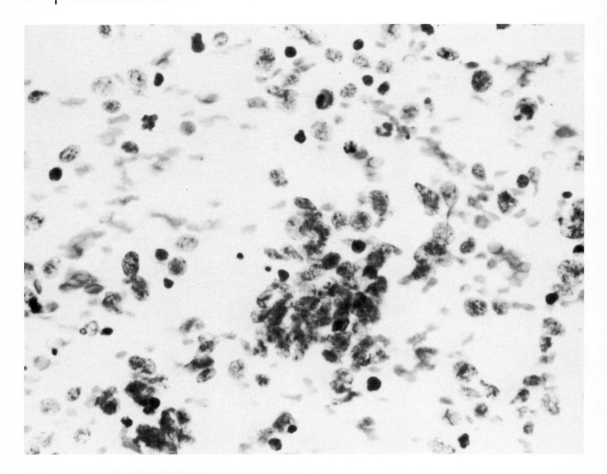

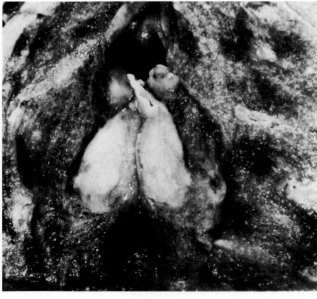

Fig. 5-61. (Above) Needle aspirate, Papanicolaou's stain, 625×, small cell undifferentiated carcinoma, oat cell type.

Fig. 5-62. (Left) Lobectomy specimen demonstrating 1 cm subpleural tumor. ⊢—⊣ = 1 cm.

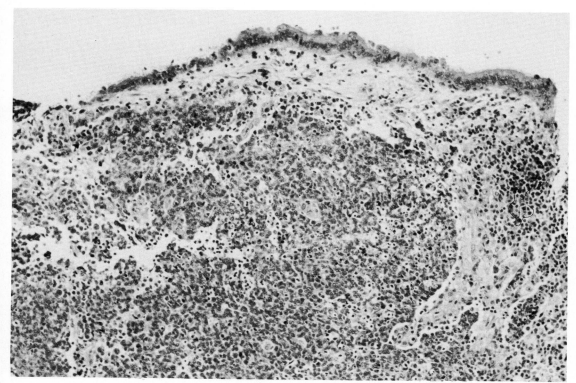

Fig. 5-63. Histological section, H&E, 160×, bronchial biopsy demonstrating oat cell carcinoma.

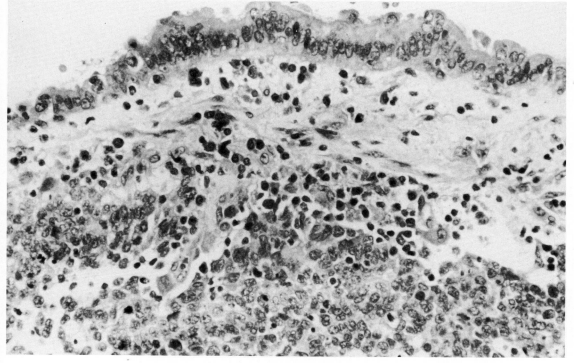

Fig. 5-64. Histological section, H&E, 400×, oat cell carcinoma.

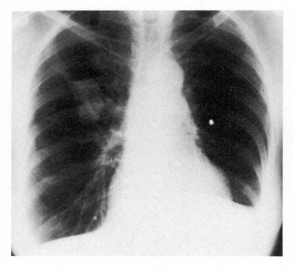

Fig. 5-65. Chest film, AP projection demonstrating mass in right upper lobe.

with focal molding of adjacent nuclei in which the chromatin was coarse and irregular. A slight tendency to spindling was noted. Silver stains disclosed characteristic granules in some cells, but origin of the tumor was not clarified.

The intermediate-sized variant of undifferentiated carcinoma is contrasted in the biopsy of a right upper lobe mass (Figs. 5-65, 5-66) from a middle-aged woman. The cells are arranged in small sheets with a semblance of polarity and with visible cytoplasm (Fig. 5-67) that occasionally exhibits definable boundaries. The almondine nuclear configurations present crisp envelopes, delicate chromatin, and prominent nucleoli. They are approximately twice the size of stimulated lymphocytes, but conform to epithelial properties. The tissue projections demonstrate spindled or oval nuclei in sheets with preserved polarity and with nuclear characteristics that repeat the texture and pattern of

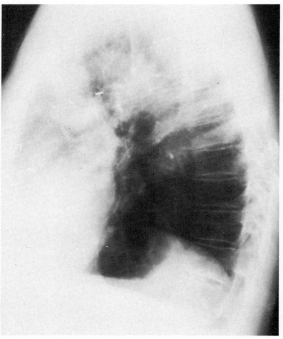

Fig. 5-66. Chest film, lateral projection accentuating mass in right upper lobe.

the aspirated cells (Fig. 5-68). If it were not for their distinctly larger size, the mimicry of oat cell carcinoma would be quite approximate.

This pattern is repeated in the aspirate investigation of a peripheral nodule in the right upper lobe of a 64-year-old woman with prior history of melanoma of the foot (Fig. 5-69a). The coin lesion was expected to represent metastatic melanoma, but the cells were small and round, with minimal cytoplasm, coarse chromatin, and indistinct nucleoli, approximating the size of lymphoblasts, but conforming to an epithelial pattern of association (Fig. 5-69b). The aspiration biopsy permitted definition of a second and separate primary cancer, and the patient was referred for lobectomy. The resected tumor resided beneath the pleura (Fig. 5-70), appeared unencapsulated with minimal variegation. The

transected surface exhibited a granular pattern without significant necrosis. Microscopically, the neoplasm was constructed of a monomorphous population of undifferentiated round epithelial cells of intermediate size in lobulated confluences (Fig. 5-71). These did not resemble the cellular constituents of the antecedent malignant melanoma.

The clinical necessity to verify metastatic dissemination from an established malignant neoplasm is implicit in the differential interpretation of a pulmonary opacification. Fine needle aspiration cytology may validate the metastatic deposit, or as in the previous case, alert the physician to the occurrence of a second, and treatable, primary tumor. In some instances, the abnormality in the x-ray may be the result of scarification or an opportunistic infection.

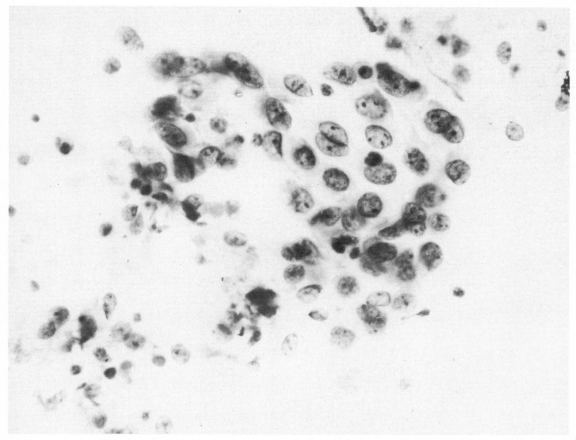

Fig. 5-67. Needle aspirate, Papanicolaou's stain, 625×, small cell undifferentiated carcinoma, intermediate cell type.

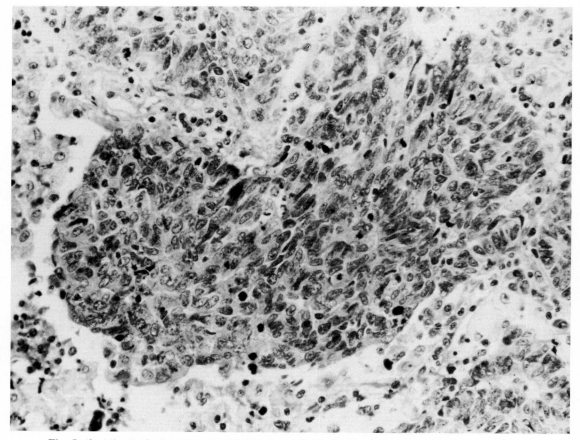

Fig. 5-68. Histological section, H&E, 400×, undifferentiated carcinoma, intermediate cell type.

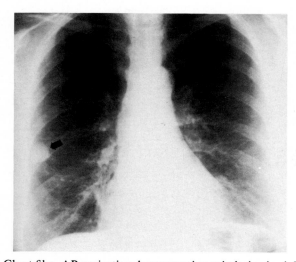

Fig. 5-69 a. Chest film, AP projection demonstrating coin lesion in right upper lobe.

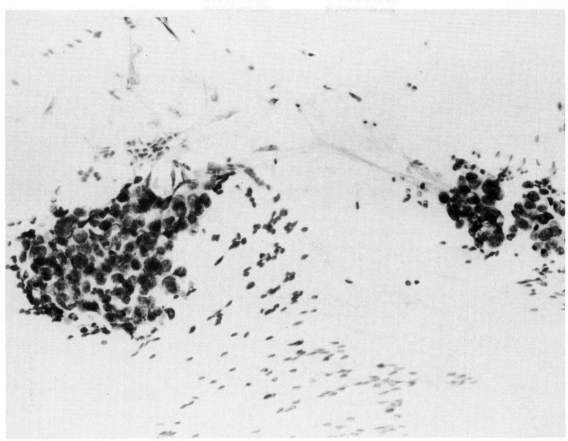

Fig. 5-69 b. Needle aspirate, Papanicolaou's stain, 315×, undifferentiated carcinoma intermediate cell type.

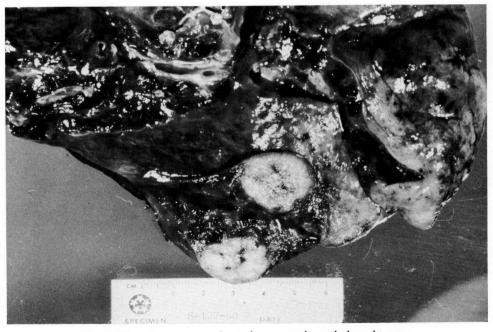

Fig. 5-70. Lobectomy specimen demonstrating subpleural tumor.

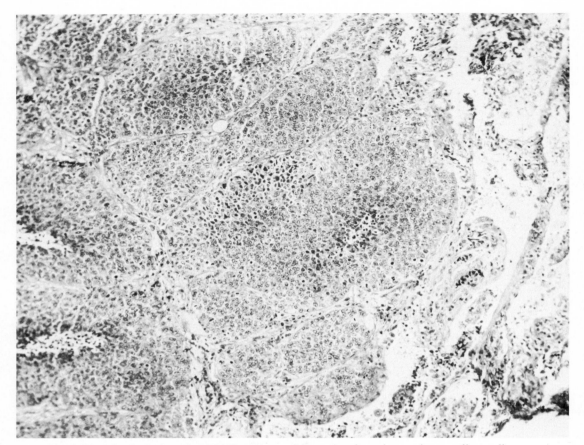

Fig. 5-71. Histological section, H&E, 125×, undifferentiated carcinoma, intermediate cell type.

The metastatic lesion can be analyzed with facility, using a conventional technique, amplified by comparison with slides of the primary specimen aspirates. A 63-year-old concert pianist presented with posterior cervical lymphadenopathy approximately 2 years following resection of a lesion from the pinna of the right ear. A lymph node biopsy was performed at another institution, review of the slides resulted in the opinion of metastatic melanoma, and a right radical neck dissection was accomplished. Approximately 1 year later, a circumscribed mass appeared in the right middle lobe (Figs. 5-72, 5-73). Aspiration biopsy was conducted under fluoroscopic control and the abundant cellular harvest consisted of polyhedral cells in loose mosaic aggregates with fusiform elements and nuclear characteristics of malignancy. The prominent nucleoli of melanoma cells were conspicuous (Fig. 5-74), but intranuclear cyto-

plasmic invaginations were not evident, and melanin granules could not be demonstrated in the cytoplasm without histochemical assistance. The cells were identical with the metastatic amelanotic melanoma retrieved from cervical lymph nodes (Fig. 5-75). Despite intensive chemotherapeutic effort, the patient expired with marrow depression and disseminated tumor.

A 74-year-old male was admitted for evaluation of a solitary nodule in the left upper lobe 6 years following tissue diagnosis of prostatic adenocarcinoma (Fig. 5-76). The lesion was fluoroscopically localized, and a 22-gauge spinal needle was used for sampling, according to conventional technique (Fig. 5-77). Columnar cells were arranged in definitive rosettes or as singly disported elements (Fig. 5-78), exhibiting enlarged, convoluted nuclei with intensification of nuclear margins by chromatin precipitation at

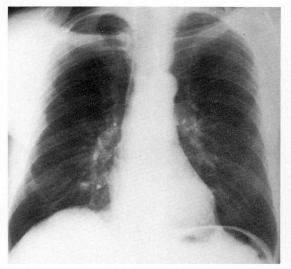

Fig. 5-72. Chest film, AP projection demonstrating lesion in right middle lobe.

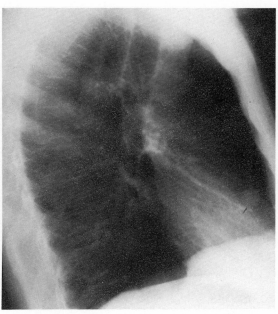

Fig. 5-73. Chest film, lateral projection demonstrating right middle lobe lesion.

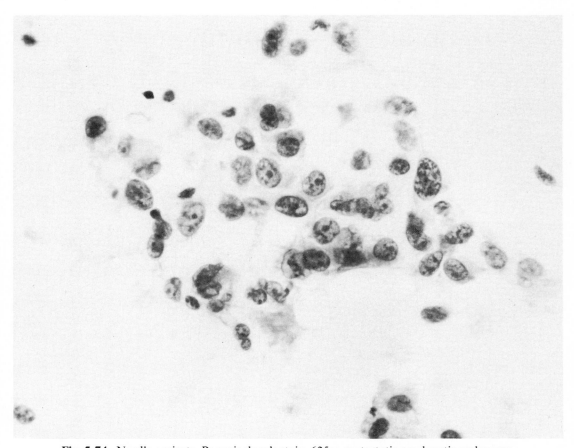

Fig. 5-74. Needle aspirate, Papanicolaou's stain, 625×, metastatic amelanotic melanoma.

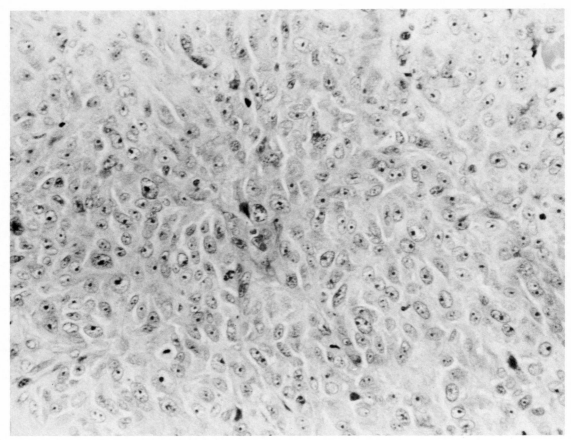

Fig. 5-75. Histological section, H&E, 400×, metastatic melanoma in cervical lymph node.

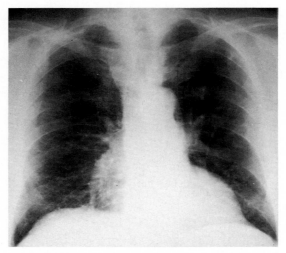

Fig. 5-76. Chest film, AP projection demonstrating mass in left upper lobe.

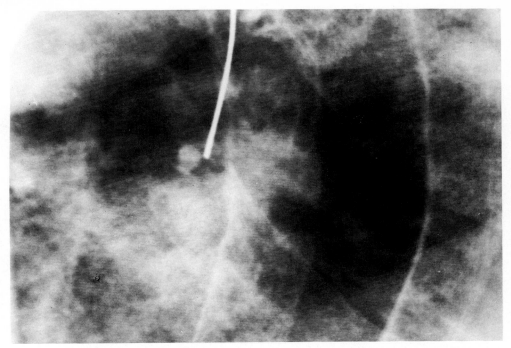

Fig. 5-77. Fluoroscopic image intensified placement of the needle is demonstrated.

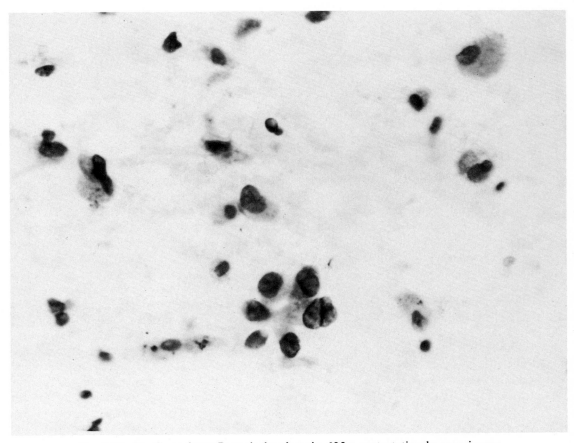

Fig. 5-78. Needle aspirate, Papanicolaou's stain, 625×, metastatic adenocarcinoma.

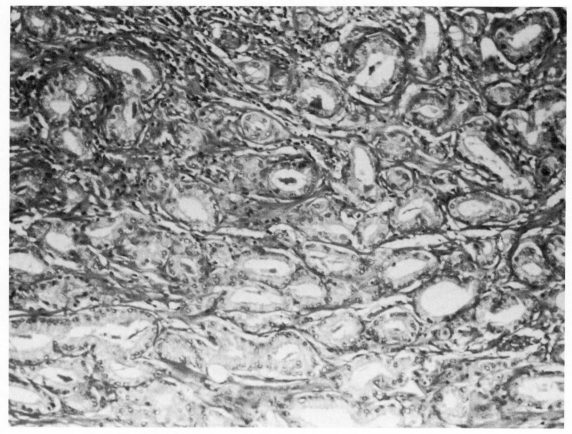

Fig. 5-79. Histological section, H&E, 400×, primary prostatic adenocarcinoma.

the periphery. Nucleoli were present, but certainly not dominant, and creases within the nuclei were accentuated by alignment of chromatin granules. The acinar arrangement of the tumor cells and their rather bland nuclear properties correlated directly with the well-differentiated acini of the primary prostatic tumor (Fig. 5-79). Lobectomy was elected because tumor was apparently confined to the solitary pulmonary deposit, which was incorporated within parenchyma as a discrete, but unencapsulated 1.2 cm gray-white mass (Fig. 5-80 a). Histological preparations demonstrated serrated glandular structures composed of cells with vesicular, bland nuclei resembling the aspirated counterparts and the primary prostatic image (Fig. 5-80 b).

A 60-year-old male was admitted for evaluation of hemoptysis. Chest roentgenography demonstrated peculiar thin-walled cystic cavities in the right upper lobe and left mid-lung field (Fig. 5-81), with the former confirmed by CAT examination of the chest (Fig. 5-82). An intermediate-strength tuberculin test was positive, and possibility of an infectious etiology was strongly contemplated. A fine needle aspirate was obtained from the right upper lobe cavity (Fig. 5-83), and demonstrated a myriad of macrophages with coarsely refractile hemosiderin granules, and conventional pneumonocytes, punctuated by bizarre spindle cells with coarsely hyperchromatic, convoluted, enlarged nuclei that occupied half the fusiform cytoplasm or distended the cytoplasmic membranes. A diagnosis of sarcoma was offered and the patient was consulted about the possibility of a prior extrapulmonary tumor. The interview contributed the information that an angiosarcoma had been excised from the scalp 2 years earlier (Fig. 5-84), and the original slides were reviewed for

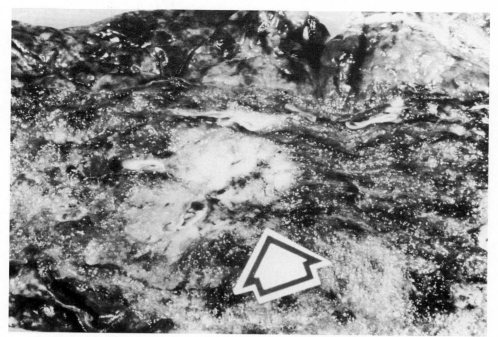

Fig. 5-80 a. Lobectomy specimen with a circumscribed, gray-white, 1.2 cm neoplasm.

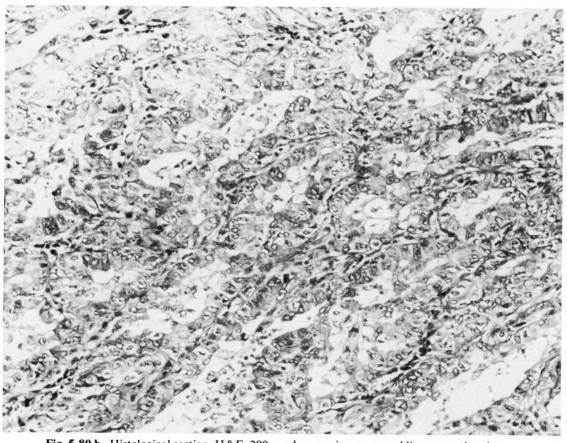

Fig. 5-80 b. Histological section, H&E, 200×, adenocarcinoma resembling prostatic primary.

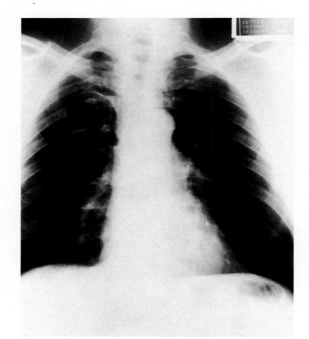

Fig. 5-81. Chest film, AP projection demonstrating thin-walled cystic mass in right upper lobe.

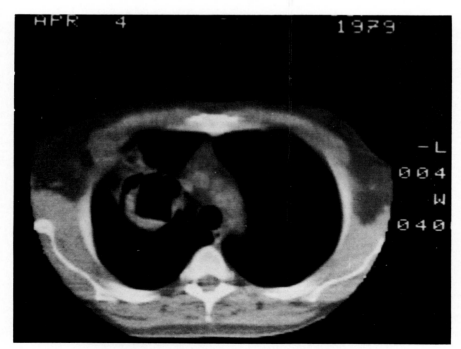

Fig. 5-82. CAT of chest demonstrating cystic mass.

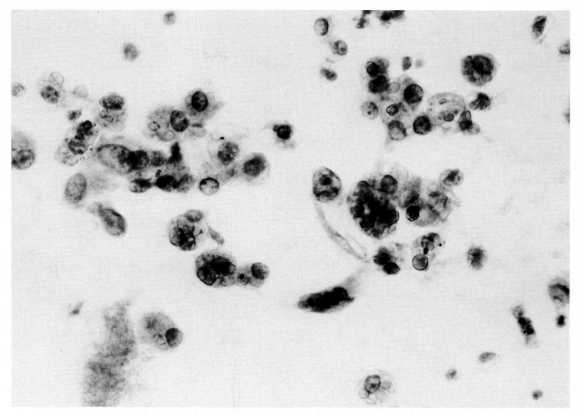

Fig. 5-83. Needle aspirate, Papanicolaou's stain, 500×, metastatic angiosarcoma.

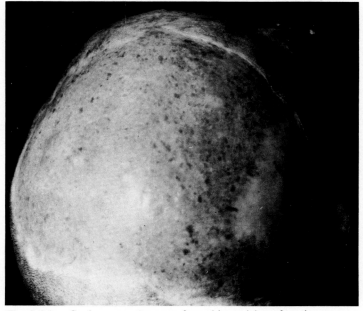

Fig. 5-84 a. Scalp, status 2 years after wide excision of angiosarcoma.

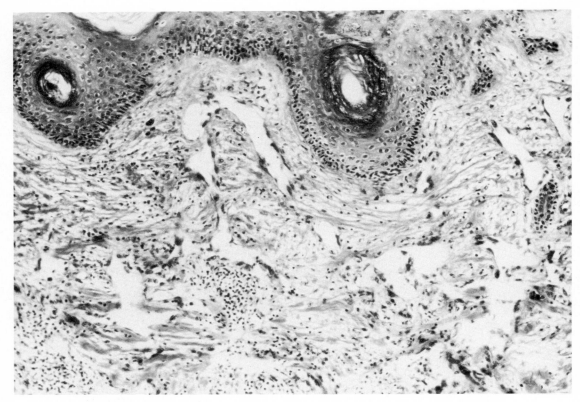

Fig. 5-84 b. Histological section, H&E, 160×, skin of scalp with primary angiosarcoma.

corroboration. These demonstrated a primary angiomatous process involving the skin of the scalp, with formidable spindle cells lining anastomosing vascular channels. Identity was established between the pulmonary aspirate population and the scalp tumor, and a diagnosis of metastatic angiosarcoma was confirmed. A metastatic survey revealed evidence for cystic lesions in the liver and a two-stage laparotomy-thoracotomy was planned. Direct examination of the hepatic cysts with biopsy disclosed metastatic angiosarcoma (Fig. 5-85), and thoracotomy was deferred, so that confirmation of the aspirate diagnosis remains indirect.

A 72-year-old male presented with left hilar adenopathy several months following a segmental bladder resection for anaplastic transitional cell carcinoma with focal squamous differentiation (Fig. 5-86). A directed aspiration biopsy obtained cells in papillary clusters and trabecular cords (Fig. 5-87). The transitional nuclei

appeared round, with crisp margins and prominent nucleoli, and were interspersed with large, polyhedral cells with coarse chromatin dispersion and suggestive pearl formation (Fig. 5-88), interpreted as correspondents to the squamoid element. Cellular identity was established between the primary bladder tumor (Fig. 5-89) and the aspirate, and ultimately confirmed by autopsy.

A 39-year-old woman presented with a stellate lesion in the left lung 11 months following modified right radical mastectomy for medullary carcinoma (Fig. 5-90). The aspirate contained only a few clusters of epithelial cells with nuclear variations (Fig. 5-91). Although a diagnosis was rendered on the basis of comparison with the histological sections of the breast mass (Fig. 5-92), this preparation is suboptimal because of inadequate numbers of cells and obscurity of nuclear detail. The cytopathologist is cautioned to demand a high quality sample and to avoid

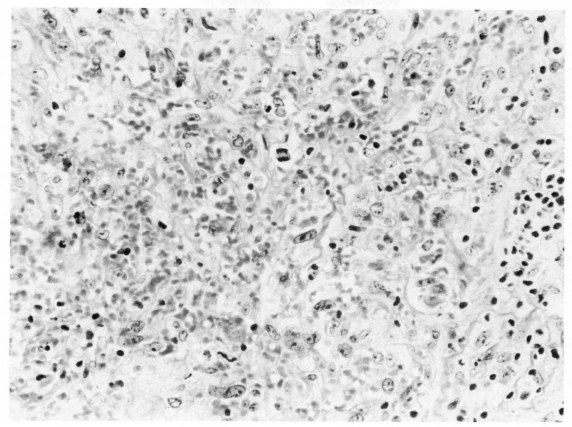

Fig. 5-85. Histological section, H&E, 400×, biopsy of hepatic cyst demonstrating metastatic angiosarcoma.

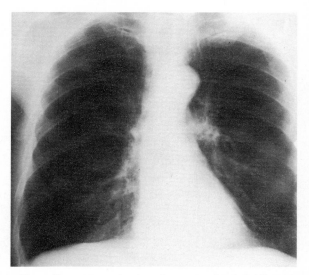

Fig. 5-86. Chest film, AP projection demonstrating left hilar adenopathy.

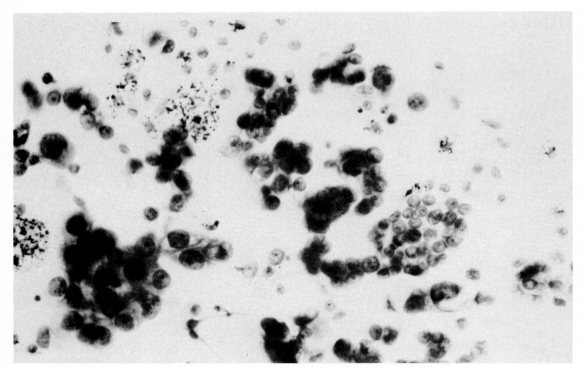

Fig. 5-87. Needle aspirate, Papanicolaou's stain, 400×, metastatic transitional cell carcinoma.

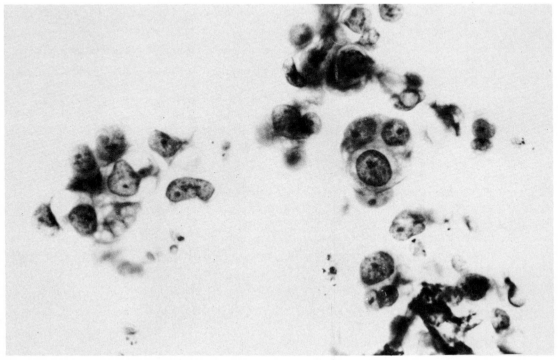

Fig. 5-88. Needle aspirate, Papanicolaou's stain, 625×, metastatic transitional cell carcinoma with squamoid features.

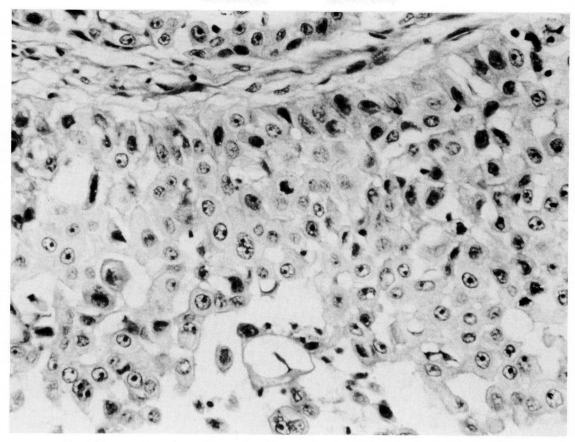

Fig. 5-89. Histological section, H&E, 400×, primary transitional cell carcinoma of bladder.

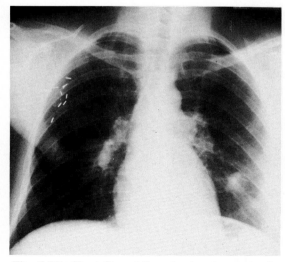

Fig. 5-90. Chest film, AP projection demonstrating mass in left lower lobe.

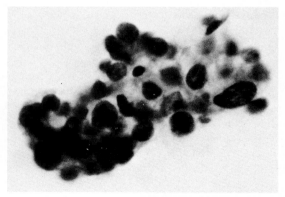

Fig. 5-91. Needle aspirate, Papanicolaou's stain, 800×, metastatic breast carcinoma demonstrating suboptimal cellular quality.

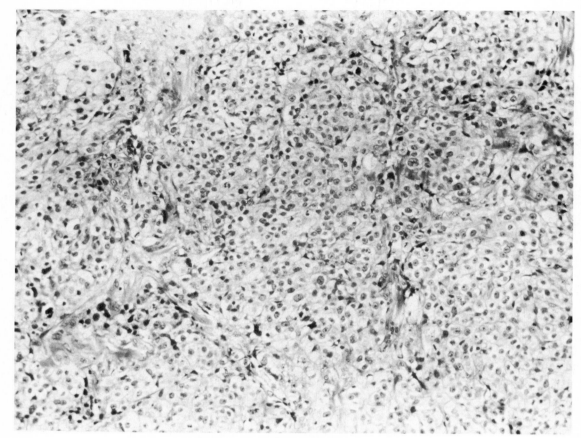

Fig. 5-92. Histological section, H&E, 200×, primary breast cancer.

heavy reliance on history, thereby avoiding interpretative compromise.

An 80-year-old male was admitted for concomitant evaluation of a left neck mass (suspected to represent a salivary gland neoplasm) and a left posterior pulmonary opacity (Fig. 5-93, 5-94). An 8 by 6 by 5 cm spherical tan mass was resected from the neck and histological studies confirmed carcinoma arising in a pleomorphic adenoma (Fig. 5-95). The hypercellularity of the proliferating epithelial component and its destructive invasive quality led to a diagnosis of a primary malignancy, and the cellular aspirate from the lung (Fig. 5-96) exhibited concordance of cellular detail. Further therapy was predicated on this information.

Our opportunity to study benign neoplasms by fine needle aspiration cytology has been regrettably limited, but one fascinating case deserves illustration. A 66-year-old male was under

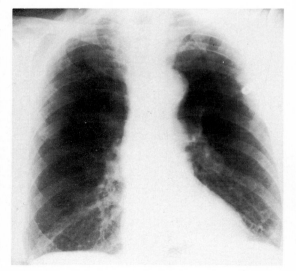

Fig. 5-93. Chest film, AP projection demonstrating left posterior lung mass.

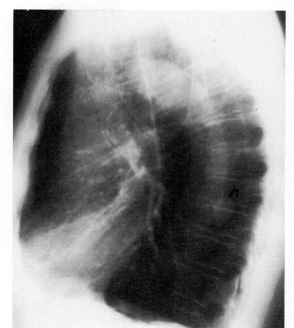

Fig. 5-94. Chest film, lateral projection demonstrating left posterior pulmonary lesion.

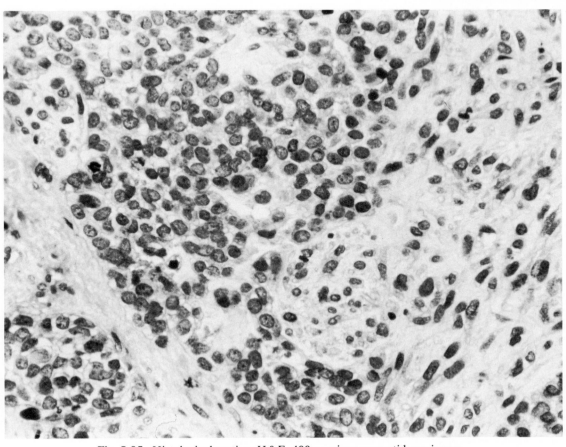

Fig. 5-95. Histological section, H & E, 400×, primary parotid carcinoma.

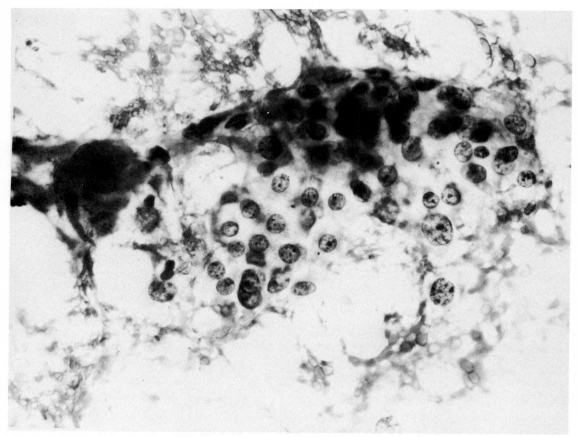

Fig. 5-96. Needle aspirate, Papanicolaou's stain, 625×, metastatic carcinoma, consistent with origin from parotid primary.

surveillance for respiratory tract infections and a persistent, apparently inert 5 cm mass at the apex of the left lung (Fig. 5-97). He had been aware of the mass for many years, and apparently there had been no change in size, or in the smooth, sharply delimited contour. A fine needle aspirate (Fig. 5-98) disclosed large, benign, occasionally binucleate polyhedral cells and blue-gray homogeneous acellular ground substance. The material was interpreted to represent a chondromatous hamartoma, an impression shared by the radiologists and clinical associates. Further investigation and excision were deferred.

DIFFUSE INFILTRATES, NODULAR INFECTIONS

Identification of a specific organism or isolation for cultural confirmation can be accom-

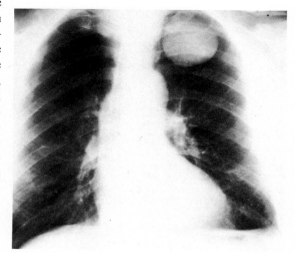

Fig. 5-97. Chest film, AP projection demonstrating well-circumscribed benign mass in left upper lobe.

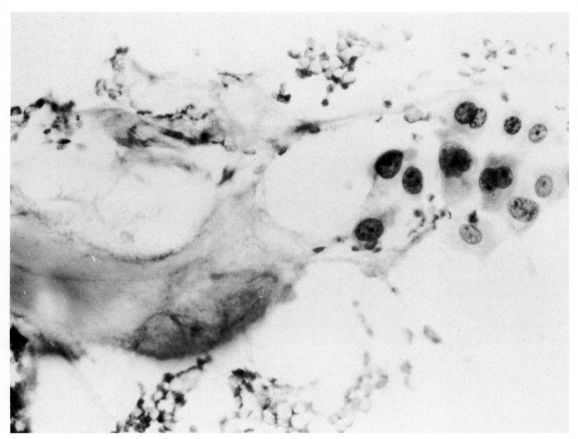

Fig. 5-98. Needle aspirate, Papanicolaou's stain, 625×, chondromatous hamartoma.

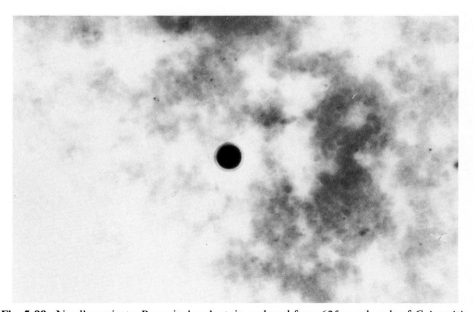

Fig. 5-99. Needle aspirate, Papanicolaou's stain, reduced from 625×, spherule of *C. immitis.*

plished atraumatically with aspiration biopsy. We are not aware of concrete evidence that infection is transmitted along the needle tract when a granuloma is penetrated, and our brief follow-up of cases in which coccidioidomycosis has been identified has not contributed information to dispute this.

The appearance of the spherule of *C. immitis* isolated by needle aspiration is indicated in Figure 5-99. A doubly refractile shell encloses endospores whose structure is obscured in this photograph. The granuloma from which the aspirate was derived is a well-circumscribed, suggestively laminated, gray-white nodule without caseation necrosis (Fig. 5-100). The histological preparation (Fig. 5-101) demonstrates the junction of granuloma with adjacent pulmonary parenchyma, and Gomori's silver methenamine stains accentuate the spherules (Fig. 5-102). The organisms are visible with Papanicolaou's stain and may be inoculated in appropriate culture media from the saline needle wash supernatant.

When the pulmonary infiltrate is not circumscribed, it is a less effective target for needle aspiration. When the process is benign and etiologically nonspecific, the cellular harvest may be similarly nondescript, and clinical confirmation of a benign cytological diagnosis requires resolution of the radiographic abnormality and symptomatology. A 62-year-old male presented with cough productive of sputum with a benign cellular population and flora. The chest film disclosed an indiscrete infiltrate in the left lower lobe (Figs. 5-103, 5-104). The needle aspirate incorporated a pure population of granular pneumonocytes in various postures of reactivity. Nuclei appeared eccentric and reniform, incorporated within abundant cytoplasm containing granules of foreign material (Fig. 5-105). No specific microorganisms were detected. The opinion of the cytopathologist was that the process was reactive, benign, and nonspecific. The patient was released to surveillance and 14 months later was asymptomatic with resolution of the infiltrate (Fig. 5-106). A 62-year-old woman was evaluated by bronchoscopy for an infiltrate in the right lower lobe (Fig. 5-107, 5-108) and benign bronchial and inflammatory cells were retrieved. A bronchial biopsy disclosed no significant atypia. The lesion was subsequently examined by needle aspiration and fibrinopurulent exudate was the product (Fig. 5-109). The material was submitted for Gram's stain and culture and no microorganisms were

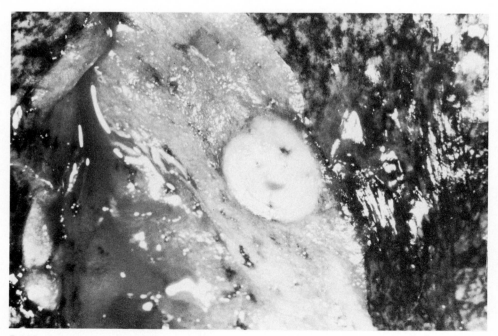

Fig. 5-100. Lobectomy specimen incorporating well-circumscribed laminated granuloma of *C. immitis.*

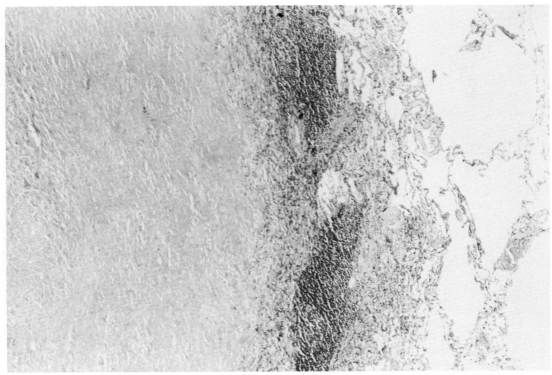

Fig. 5-101. Histological section, H&E, 62.5×, granuloma of *C. immitis.*

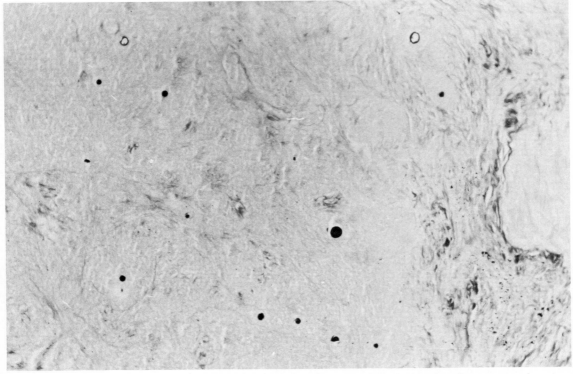

Fig. 5-102. Histological section, Gomori's silver methenamine, 160×, spherules of *C. immitis.*

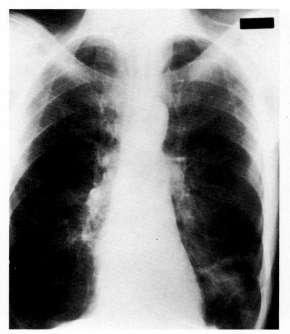

Fig. 5-103. Chest film, AP projection demonstrating poorly defined infiltrate in left lower lobe.

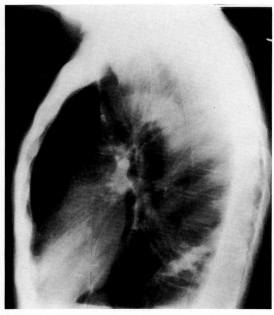

Fig. 5-104. Chest film, lateral projection demonstrating poorly defined infiltrate, left lower lobe.

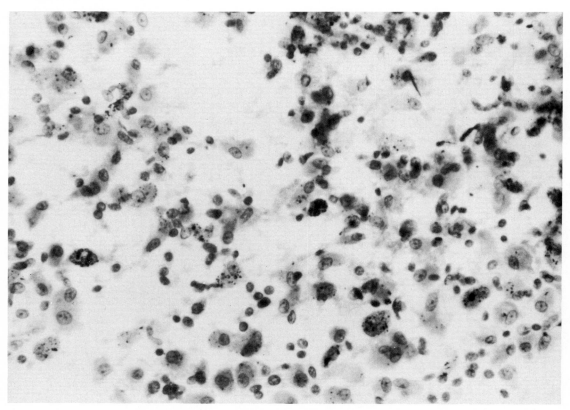

Fig. 5-105. Needle aspirate, Papanicolaou's stain, 400×, reactive pneumonocytes and inflammatory cells.

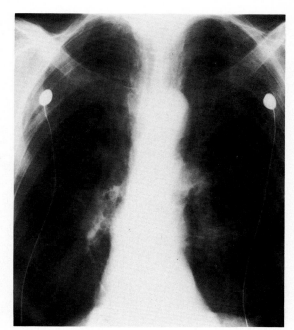

Fig. 5-106. Chest film, AP projection, resolution of pulmonary infiltrate.

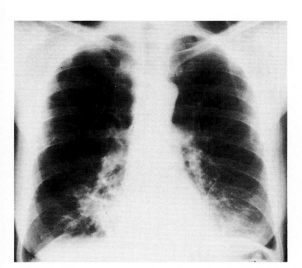

Fig. 5-107. Chest film, right lower lobe infiltrate.

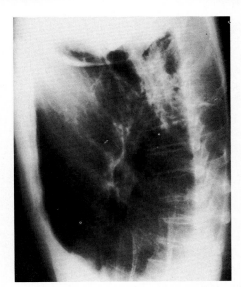

Fig. 5-108. Chest film, lateral projection, right lower lobe infiltrate.

detected. A diagnosis of sterile abscess was offered. A benign diagnosis by aspiration of a vague infiltrate is somewhat unsatisfying because further intervention may be deferred to surveillance, and confirmation resides in the abstract resolution of a process too ethereal to be captured by biopsy for perpetuation on slides.

The results are rewarding when a specific etiological agent is encountered and the patient recovers. If there is a high clinical index of suspicion for a malignant process, a benign aspiration does not exclude cancer and further investigation is mandated.

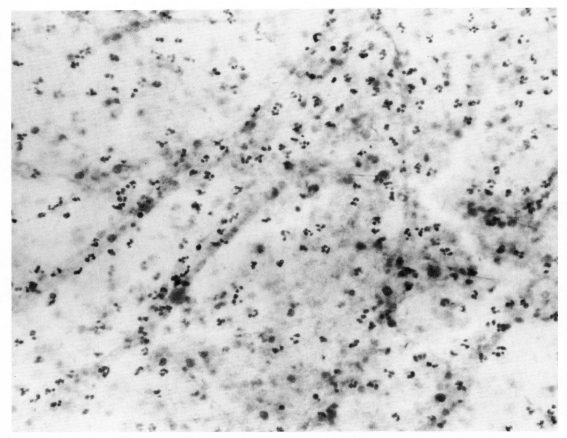

Fig. 5-109. Needle aspirate, Papanicolaou's stain, 400×, fibrinopurulent exudate, consistent with origin from abscess.

REFERENCES

1. Fontana, R. S., Miller, W. E., Beabout, J. W., Payne, W. S., and Harrison, E. G.: Transthoracic needle aspiration of discrete pulmonary lesions: Experience in 100 cases. *Med Clin North Am* **54**(4): 961–971, 1970.
2. Stevens, G. M., Weigen, J. F., and Lillington, G. A.: Needle aspiration biopsy of localized pulmonary lesions with amplified fluoroscopic guidance. *AJR* **103**(3): 561–571, 1968.
3. Dahlgren, S. E., and Lind, B.: Comparison between diagnostic results obtained by transthoracic needle biopsy and by sputum cytology. *Acta Cytol* **16**(1): 53–58, 1972.
4. Dahlgren, S. E., and Nordenstrom, B.: *Transthoracic Needle Biopsy.* Almqvist & Wiksells, Stockholm, 1966.
5. Johnston, W. W., and Frable, W. J.: *Diagnostic Respiratory Cytopathology.* Masson Publishing USA, New York, 1979.
6. Pavy, R. D., Antic, R., and Begley, M.: Percutaneous aspiration biopsy of discrete lung lesions. *Cancer* **34**: 2109–2117, 1974.
7. Zornoza, J., Snow, J., Lukeman, J. M., and Libshitz, H. I.: Aspiration biopsy of discrete pulmonary lesion using a new thin needle. *Work Prog* **123**: 519–520, 1977.
8. Meyer, J. E., Gandbhir, L. H., Milner, L. B., and McLaughlin, M. M.: Percutaneous aspiration biopsy of nodular lung lesions. *J Thorac Cardiovasc Surg* **73**: 787–791, 1977.
9. Landman, S., Burgener, F. A., and Lim, G. H. K.: Comparison of bronchial brushing and percutaneous needle aspiration biopsy in the diagnosis of malignant lung lesions. *Radiology* **115**: 275–278, 1975.
10. Sinner, W. N.: Transthoracic needle biopsy of small peripheral malignant lung lesions. *Invest Radiol* **8**(5): 305–314, 1973.
11. Milner, L. B., Ryan, K., and Gullo, J.: Fatal intrathoracic hemorrhage after percutaneous aspiration lung biopsy. *AJR* **132**: 280–281, 1979.
12. Zelch, J. V., and Lalli, A. F.: Diagnostic percutaneous opacification of benign pulmonary lesions. *Radiology* **108**: 559–561, 1973.
13. Sinner, W. N., and Sandstedt, B.: Small-cell carcinoma of the lung. *Radiology* **121**: 269–274, 1976.

Computed Axial Tomography in the Selection of Cell Samples from Abdominal Masses

Technical Descriptions and Radiologic Applications by Joel H. Thayer, M.D.

The advent of CAT has revolutionized the identification and localization of intra-abdominal space-occupying lesions and introduced a sophisticated mechanism to insure the precise placement of the thin biopsy needle for aspiration of cellular samples. The coordination of the diagnostic radiologist and cytopathologist in the selection of the biopsy site and in the guidance of the needle to target has resulted in a rapid, precise, cost-effective method, at minimal risk to the patient, for establishing primary malignancy, metastatic dissemination or inflammatory disease within the abdomen. The test may be performed on an outpatient basis, avoid costly hospitalization, and can obviate exploratory laparotomy. This is of particular value and applicability to the elderly or high risk patient with presumptive malignancy, for whom surgical intervention is contraindicated, but who requires definitive diagnosis prior to the initiation of radiotherapy or systemic chemotherapy. Our experience with aspiration biopsy of the liver, pancreas, pelvis, and retroperitoneum reiterates the opinions of Haaga and Alfidi[1] of the Cleveland Clinic that "localization by computed tomography is the single most accurate method for performing biopsies."

TECHNICAL DESCRIPTIONS AND RADIOLOGIC APPLICATIONS

Computerized Axial Tomography: History and Historical Aspects

Conventional radiographic recording techniques have changed very little since Roentgen's original work. For tissue interfaces where considerable density differences exist, for example within chest, plain radiographic techniques have been superb. In areas of the body where soft tissues predominate, for example within abdomen or within the intracranial vault, plain radiographs are insensitive to the relatively small differences in tissue radiodensity. Techniques using contrast media have provided some improvement in changing differential tissue density, although for enhancement of intracranial components, intra-arterial injection of contrast via angiography has usually been used, resulting in higher morbidity.

Using preliminary research compiled by Oldendorf, Kuhl, and Edwards, Godfrey Hounsfield,[2] a research physicist for the EMI corporation of Sussex, England, developed a prototype CAT scanner in 1971. Since the first unit was installed in the United States in 1973, this new modality has revolutionized the noninvasive diagnostic imaging field.

Technique

The principle of CAT is based upon scanning the head or other body parts using a beam of x-rays in a series of contiguous slices. Each slice is x-rayed circumferentially and the degree of x-ray attenuation by tissues traversed by the beam is measured from many directions.[3] Current CAT units are based on one of two basic principles: (1) Rotate-translate, or (2) rotating pulsed-fan beam array.

Rotate-Translate Principle. First and second generation EMI scanners are based on the rotate-translate principle. In this type of scanner, (Fig. 6-1) the patient is studied by multiple narrow x-ray beams emitted by a single x-ray tube. The beam is detected by 30 or more sensitive detectors that are positioned in diametric opposition to a single x-ray tube. All components are fixed on a common frame. Tightly collimated x-ray beams measure between 3 and 16 mm according to the type of collimater (beam restrictor) used. As the x-ray beam passes through tissues on the way to the detector system, it is absorbed in proportion to the traversed tissue density in the x-ray path. A tremendous number of x-ray density readings ranging between 15 to 50,000, depending on the scan program, are recorded by the detectors during each linear pass, each pass requiring 1 second. Upon completion of a single pass, the scanner frame rotates a predetermined number of degrees, for example, 10°, and repeats the linear traverse pass recording another slice of data. This rotate-translate procedure continues around the body until a total of 180° has been completed. Total scan time is variable, depending upon the scanner; however, average total scan time ranges between 10 and 20 seconds per slice.

The individual density readings obtained during each linear traverse are digitalized to a computer system. One or more computers are used to integrate and display the several thousand absorption readings obtained during scanning. The displays produced by the computers are usually presented on a viewing screen mounted on a convenient console (Fig. 6-2). Polaroid or multiformat x-ray prints are then exposed from the viewing screen image (Fig.

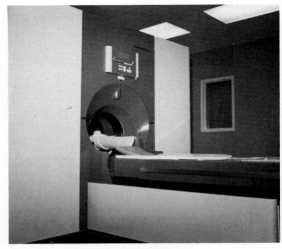

Fig. 6-1. The EMI scanner.

6-3). The more sophisticated scanners now available are capable of resolving areas of less than 1 sq. ml.

Pulsed Fan X-ray Beam. Shorter scanning time can generally be obtained by using a different scanning principle, the pulsed fan x-ray beam. This system involves a continuous 360° rotation of the x-ray tube around the scanned body part with diametrically opposed detectors. Rather than a pencil thin beam as is used in rotate-translate scanners, a pulsed fan-shaped x-ray beam is generated that passes through the desired tissue level and is recorded by an array of 600 or more separate detectors. The entire body section scanned is always within the confines of the x-ray fan beam. Scan time for each body slice obtained by this method may be as short as 5–10 seconds rather than the 20 seconds scan time required by rotate-translate units.

Factors That Degrade and Enhance Image Quality. Motion of any sort causes artifacts on CAT scans. In body scanning, the advent of fast scanners using pulsed beam technology has decreased the artifacts caused by respiratory motion; however, peristalsis, vascular pulsation, and actual patient movement remain problems. Glucagon or atropinic drugs can be given to temporarily diminish peristalsis. Parenteral sedation may diminish patient motion when reassurance about the procedure does not produce full cooperation. Vascular motion is

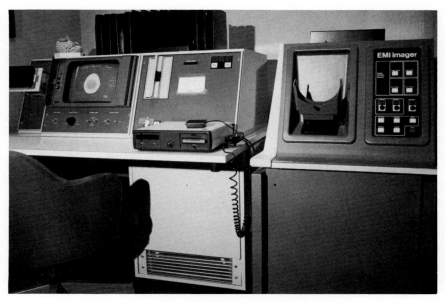

Fig. 6-2. Viewing console.

unavoidable with current equipment, although in the future scanners used for thoracic scanning are likely to be gaited with the electrocardiogram to diminish cardiac pulsation. At present, all thoracic scanning has some motion in image degradation.[4,5]

Other causes of image degradation include artifacts, such as retained barium, metallic surgical clips, or prostheses. In general, any high density object is likely to cause artifacts when included in the plane of scan. Another source of artifact not directly related to the scanned object is the computer program itself. For example, extremity scans frequently have artifacts caused by unusual distribution of air and bone. The computer is not programmed to accept this distribution and usually produces a spray or circular artifact. The computerized tomographic principle works best in situations in which the absorption values of the diseased tissues are

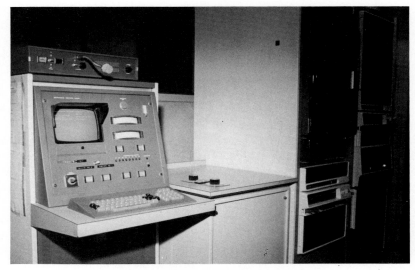

Fig. 6-3. Central computer operations.

significantly different from those of surrounding normal tissues. On standard video displays, high density lesions that have greater absorption values appear as white areas, whereas low density lesions that have lower absorption values appear as black areas. Contrast media are frequently used in CAT head and body scanning. In head scanning, intravenous iodinated contrast media increases the absorption values of well-vascularized lesions and thus allows the detection of small lesions not normally identifiable on noncontrast scans, since intrinsic nonenhanced absorption values of pathological tissue may not differ greatly from surrounding normal tissue.[6] Water soluble contrast material administered orally is used in CAT body scanning for gastric and small bowel opacification.[7] This is often of value in body scanning in order to differentiate bowel from adjacent normal or abnormal structures. Nonopacified bowel loops can often be confused with masses or enlarged lymph nodes. All barium-based contrast materials are too dense for this purpose. Intravenous contrast material is used in body scanning to identify blood vessels, to locate the ureters, and to enhance attenuation differences between normal and abnormal tissues. Oral and intravenous gall-bladder contrast agents are sometimes used for study of the biliary system. Dilute water soluble contrast media or air may be given by rectum if it is necessary to identify or distend the large bowel.

Patient Positioning for Scanning.

Most units are capable of scanning patients in supine, prone, and decubitis positions. Supine position is used for routine scanning.[5] Prone and decubitis are usually reserved for specialized situations, for example, percutaneous thin needle aspiration biopsy. The number of scans in an examination is variable, depending upon the type of scan performed and the clinical questions to be answered. Most scanners have a slice thickness of about 1 cm, and therefore for brain scanning, eight to nine sections are usually adequate for a complete study. The number of scans required in body scanning is variable and usually related to patient body size and the clinical questions to be answered.[8–11]

Radiologic Thin Needle Aspiration Biopsy in Diagnosis of Malignancy

Suspected masses, whether related to a specific organ or anatomical compartment, may be diagnosed by thin needle biopsy provided they are either palpable or detectable by available imaging techniques. Small tumors in deep intra-abdominal or retroperitoneal locations require patient cooperation for positioning and breath holding; inability to cooperate is therefore a relative contraindication for small deep lesions. Contraindications are few and include bleeding diathesis and vascular primary liver tumors, including hemangioma and hepatocellular carcinoma. Vascular hepatic secondary tumors are usually biopsied without difficulty.[12]

Technique. Percutaneous aspiration biopsy is best performed with a 22- or 23-gauge Chiba needle. The tumor target mass is first localized with the simplest imaging modality that delineates the target volume. Multiple imaging modalities are available and include ultrasound;[13,14] computerized tomography;[1,15] fluoroscopy with or without contrast;[16,17] lymphangiography;[18,19] direct cholangiography;[20] endoscopic retrograde pancreatography;[21] and angiography.[22] Ultrasound or CAT localization methods have currently supplanted most other imaging modalities in abdominal fine needle biopsy diagnosis.

Patient Preparation. Minimal patient preparation is required. Blood clotting time (qualitative) and prothrombin time are usually sufficient. Fasting 4 hours prior to procedure is advisable but not always appropriate, depending on the biopsy site. For medicolegal purposes, an informed consent should be obtained. Sedation is optional, depending on physician discretion.

Equipment Needed for Guided Biopsy. A typical biopsy kit (Fig. 6-4) includes the following: (1) Suction syringe, 20 cc, (2) 22-gauge biopsy needles of varying lengths, (3) glass slides, (4) coplin jar with 95% ethanol, (5) antiseptic swabs, (6) Xylocaine, (7) needle and syringe for local anesthetic, (8) sterile drapes and sponges, (9) sterile measuring tape or ruler, (10) set screw needle stops (optional), and (11) sterile

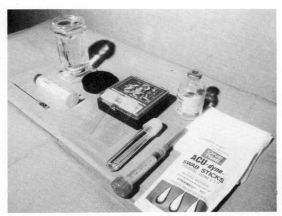

Fig. 6-4. Required implements for CT scan directed fine needle aspiration of abdominal masses.

mineral oil and transducer (ultrasound guidance only).

Biopsy Procedure. *Step One.* Locate the target of the biopsy using the chosen imaging modality (Fig. 6-5).

Step Two. Choose the needle entry site and trajectory. This is usually the shortest distance from skin to the mass. The optimal needle trajectory is usually perpendicular to the target mass; however, some lesion locations may not be readily biopsied unless angled trajectory is used, such as liver tumors beneath the dome of the diaphragm. Reasonable attempt is made to avoid bowel, major vessels, or nontarget organs if this does not greatly increase the distances; however, many thin needle biopsies have been performed through a nontarget solid organ or bowel with no undue affects.

Step Three. Measure the target depth distance, that is, the distance from the puncture site to the middle of the mass using the preliminary scan images.

When using ultrasound as the imaging mode, the transducer is moved until it is directly over the puncture site on the patient's skin. This is located by observing the main bang echo on the video monitor. The transducer is then removed and the puncture site marked with an "X" on the skin. The skin-to-target distance is then marked on video using manual or electronic calipers.

When using CAT as the imaging mode, the

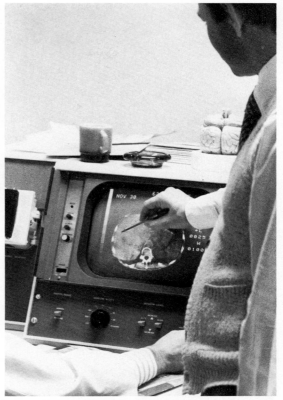

Fig. 6-5. Clinician and radiologist locate the target of the biopsy.

tandem needle maneuver is especially useful.[23] This method uses an initial "guide" or "marker" thin Chiba needle, which is positioned into the target mass and left in place. One or more additional thin needles are then passed in tandem over the sentry needle at a similar depth. This assures accurate access to the original target site without the need for repeated time-consuming CAT imaging and provides a constant reference point for multiple biopsies taken from different portions of a tumor. The alternate method, demonstrated pictorially, utilizes a single needle with repeat imaging for verification of position. The choice is a prerogative of the radiologist and varies with his training and experience.

Step Four. Following sterile preparation (Fig. 6-6), appropriate draping about the puncture site, and local anesthesia (Fig. 6-7), the needle is advanced into the lesion to a predeter-

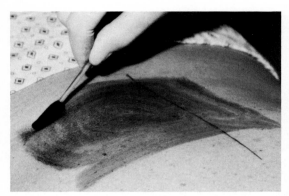

Fig. 6-6. The skin is prepared for draping with an antiseptic solution.

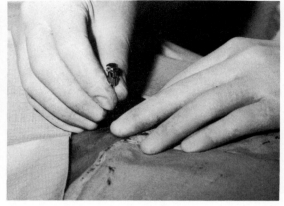

Fig. 6-9. The needle is adjusted.

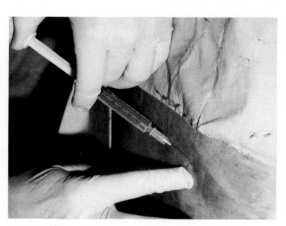

Fig. 6-7. The local anesthetic is injected.

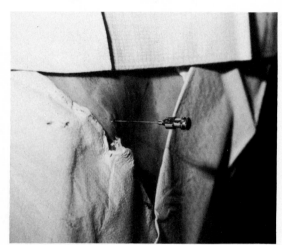

Fig. 6-10. The appropriate depth is obtained.

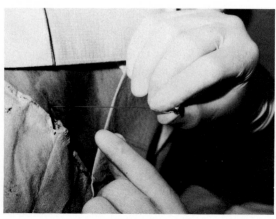

Fig. 6-8. The initial puncture is made.

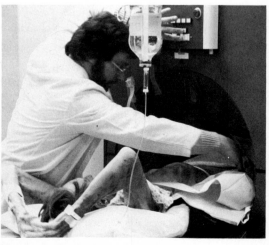

Fig. 6-11. CAT technologist, Tom Tracia, positions the patient for a scan reading to determine placement of needle.

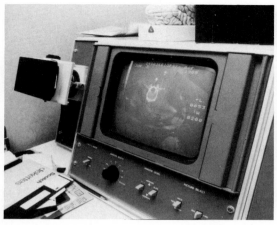

Fig. 6-12. The position of the needle is transmitted to the console viewer.

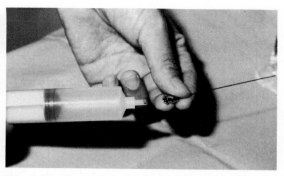

Fig. 6-15. The pathologist disconnects the needle and aspirates air into the syringe for an expulsive force to express the aspirated material onto glass slides.

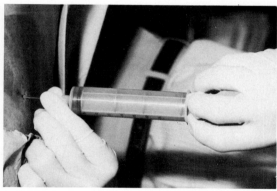

Fig. 6-13. The syringe is attached to the needle following CT scan validation of the needle tip in its target.

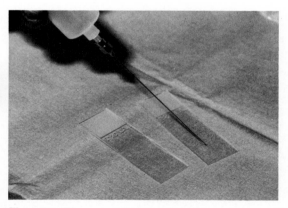

Fig. 6-16. The material is transferred from the core of the needle to one end of the glass slide.

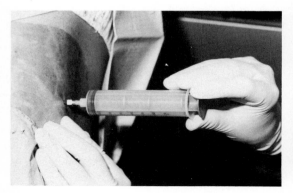

Fig. 6-14. Suction is applied and the oscillation maneuver initiated.

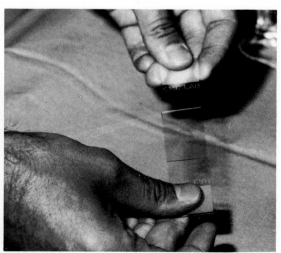

Fig. 6-17. Dispersement in a localized circular monolayer is achieved by contact of two slides without a smearing motion.

mined depth (Figs. 6-8, 6-9, 6-10). When using ultrasound imaging, sterile mineral oil and a sterile transducer must be employed.[24] Needle advancement can usually be implemented in one step. If CAT imaging is used, the initial needle tip portion is verified with serial scans through the target mass (Figs. 6-11, 6-12). Adjustments are often necessary for optimal positioning, and breath holding during needle advancement is advised.

Step Five (Obtaining the Aspirate). The stylet is removed from the biopsy needle and a suction syringe is attached to the needle positioned in its target (Fig. 6-13). Suction is applied and the needle is gently and rapidly oscillated three or four times within the confines of the mass (Fig. 6-14). Suction is released and the biopsy needle removed. The patient should be breath holding during the aspiration, which should require no more than 5 seconds.

Step 6 (Slide Preparation). The needle and syringe are transferred to the pathologist who disconnects the needle (Fig. 6-15) and aspirates air into the syringe barrel to serve as an expulsive force to express the aspirated material onto one end of a glass slide (Fig. 6-16). A second slide is placed in contact with the material until there is dispersement in a localized circular monolayer (Fig. 6-17). The slides are separated in a perpendicular direction to avoid artifact of smearing and are immediately immersed in 95% ethanol for a minimum of 5 minutes for rapid fixation. They are then stained by a rapid variant of Papanicolaou's technique. The stylet may be replaced within the lumen of the needle to express additional material, and a saline wash of the needle can be done to provide a reservoir for additional cytological material or for inoculation of culture media for identification of acid-fast bacilli and fungi. More than one pass may be necessary to obtain adequate material, and the patient should be maintained in position on the platform until the adequacy of the sample is validated. This should require ten to fifteen minutes of the technologist's time for staining and preliminary screening. The amount of specimen obtained on any single pass depends on the nature of the mass; pancreatic tumors, for example, are often very hard and only scant material

may be obtained, while a vascular tumor may yield a copious quantity of material. If the initial pass yields little or no specimen, more vigorous suction and needle oscillation should be performed on the next pass. Conversely, if the initial specimen is exclusively bloody, less suction and oscillatory movement are needed on the next attempt. In general, excess blood makes it more difficult for the cytopathologist to interpret the specimen.

Choice of Image Guidance System

Ferrucci,[12] has reported improved diagnostic accuracy for abdominal malignancy with CAT guidance (91%) compared with ultrasound with or without contrast-aided fluoroscopy (76%). In general, larger lesions (75 cm) can be readily imaged with ultrasound or contrast-aided fluoroscopy, while smaller lesions (15 cm) are better imaged with CAT. B-scan ultrasound provides a rapid and flexible approach to tumor localization. Longitudinal, transverse, and oblique scanning planes can often be easily obtained. Skin puncture site, needle trajectory and target depth can be readily determined from video or hard copy images; measured depth for tumor sampling can be directly transposed to the biopsy needle using a sterile ruler.

Unfortunately, ultrasound imaging has some limitations that must be taken into consideration. First, conventional B-scan machinery with articulated scanning arms are often unable to image the exact needle tip position constantly. This becomes important when biopsy involves small solid or even cystic lesions. The new generation of high resolution real-time transducer systems holds promise for improved imaging in this regard.[24]

The second limitation relates to the potential image degradation from overlying bowel gas. Adequate imaging of an abdominal lesion on initial examination does not guarantee adequate imaging on the day of biopsy. Obviously, ultrasound has little or no role in localizing parenchymal lung lesions.

Finally, skin access problems, such as incisions, ostomies, and tubes, often preclude adequate imaging with conventional ultrasound equipment.

Despite these acknowledged shortcomings, ultrasound is the preferred initial imaging modality because of simplicity and lack of ionizing radiation.

CAT imaging offers consistent, excellent resolution of tumor target volume and surrounding anatomical structures,[1,15,21] both for superficial and deep body locations. In addition, the needle tip can be consistently identified and therefore guided accurately into the tumor; this is especially advantageous for small deep lesions.[25] Despite these obvious advantages, CAT is limited to transverse scanning plane and longer procedure time needed for scan processing during initial and successive needle passes. Thus, practical considerations of speed and flexibility often make ultrasound the preferred guidance technique whenever the lesion can be imaged sufficiently for biopsy.

Other Imaging Modalities. Guidance using fluoroscopy with or without contrast (administered by mouth, needle, or catheter) has many biopsy applications, depending on the organ or area to be biopsied. Examples include transhepatic cholangiography, T-tube or transcatheter cholangiography, and lymphangiography.[26] Often, a combination of imaging techniques, for example, ultrasound and fluoroscopy, provide additional biopsy precision.

Postbiopsy Precautions. Little follow-up of the patient is required. Total absence of any serious side effects in large series of patients both in the United States and Europe has been recorded for abdominal thin needle biopsy. Inpatients should receive hourly vital signs for 4 hours and a hematocrit 24 hours postprocedure. Outpatients are best handled by scheduling an overnight hospital admission following biopsy.

Complications. The over-all complication rate is low in all published series ranging from 1–3%. There has been no mortality. Serious morbidity is rare and includes infection,[2] needle tract seeding with tumor,[27–35] and significant bleeding.[2] All have been reported as isolated occurrences, and most involved biopsies with needles larger than 22 gauge or involved 10 biopsy passes or more.

In summary, percutaneous fine needle aspiration is an accurate, safe, and widely applicable method for pathological diagnosis of somatic neoplasms. Although the early diagnosis may not change the over-all outcome in the cancer patient, it often obviates the need for extensive hospital tests and even exploratory surgery. It is reasonable to predict that in the future diagnostic assessment of somatic masses will include an attempt at fine needle aspiration biopsy as a routine preoperative maneuver.

ASPIRATIONS FROM PANCREATIC AND RETROPERITONEAL LESIONS

Fine needle aspiration biopsy of the pancreas under direct visualization at laparotomy has been a reliable substitute for conventional and large-bore needle biopsy, achieving an accuracy of 94% while avoiding complications of hemorrhage, fistula, pancreatitis, and death.[36] When the patient's age or medical risk status precludes exploratory laparotomy, or when dissemination as assessed by clinical and radiographic methods precludes resection, biopsy confirmation of tumor by CAT guidance is indicated. The brief clinical summaries that follow illustrate the facility with which a cytological diagnosis is ascertained by this technique. The method may be extended to sample the retroperitoneum.

An 87-year old male presented with progressive inanition, anorexia, weakness, and general deterioration complicated by sideroblastic anemia and chronic atrial fibrillation. A palpable abdominal mass was localized by CAT to the pancreas, but the patient was not considered a candidate for exploratory laparotomy. It was elected to biopsy the mass with a 22-gauge flexible spinal needle through a transthoracic approach. Despite artifact, which extends the image of the needle, the scan projections assured the appropriate localization of the needle tip within the mass (Fig. 6-18), and transit through the stomach was of no consequence. The cellular population harvested by this effort consisted of arbitrary clusters in which epithelial elements appeared dissociated. Polyhedral or columnar silhouettes embraced nuclei of variable size with coarse chromatin precipitation centrally and at the rim of the nuclear envelopes (Fig. 6-19). Nucleoli were irregular, central, and blatant. A diagnosis of pancreatic adenocarcinoma was

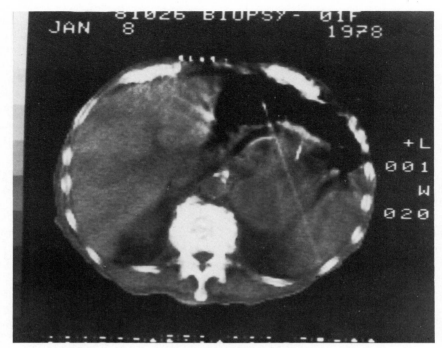

Fig. 6-18. CAT scan; transthoracic approach; needle tip in pancreatic mass.

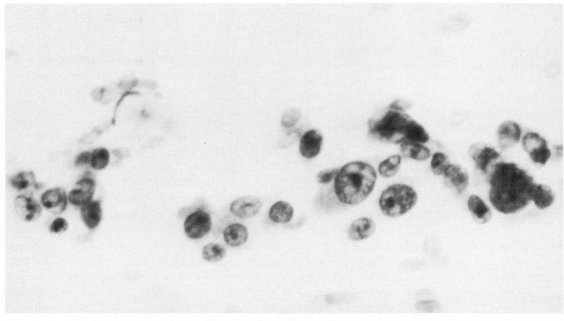

Fig. 6-19. Needle aspirate, Papanicolaou's stain, 625×, adenocarcinoma of pancreas.

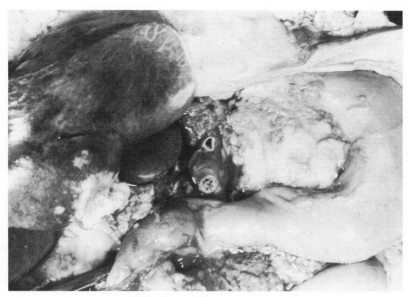

Fig. 6-20. Pancreatic mass at autopsy.

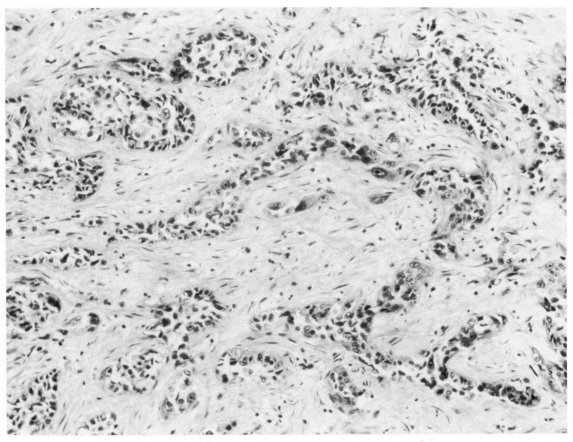

Fig. 6-21. Histological section, H&E, 200×, adenocarcinoma of pancreas.

established, and single-agent chemotherapy with 5-fluorouracil was initiated. The patient continued to deteriorate and eventually an autopsy was obtained for confirmation. A neoplasm measuring 10 cm in diameter replaced the body and tail of the pancreas and deflected the stomach anterolaterally (Fig. 6-20). It extended by direct contiguity into the splenic hilum, posterior surface of the stomach, the superior pole of the left kidney, and the left adrenal gland. Distant metastases involved the left lung. Histological sections demonstrated malignant epithelial cells arranged in bifurcating acini (Fig. 6-21). The aspirate had successfully characterized the lesion.

McLoughlin[37] reported the experience with percutaneous fine needle aspiration biopsy of malignant lesions in and around the pancreas following radiological localization. Biopsy was performed in 28 patients, a malignant diagnosis ascertained in 23, with correlative positive biopsy in 19 of the 23 (83%), including 16 of 18 patients with carcinoma of the pancreas (89%). No false positives were reported and the only complication was acute pancreatitis localized to the area circumscribing an ampullary carcinoma. Encouraging references compared the long-term survival of patients who had needle aspiration biopsies with a control group that did not, and no significant difference in survival or adverse affect on the 5-year-survival rate was noted.

An 80-year-old woman with a history and medical risk status comparable to the previous case was evaluated by CAT scan directed needle aspiration of an enlarged pancreas (Fig. 6-22). The cellular population was a suboptimal sample based on paucity of elements and deterioration with cytoplasmic degradation. However, the variability in nuclear size, shape, and chromatinic texture superimposed on a background of diathesis, provided cellular evidence of malignancy (Figs. 6-23, 6-24). At autopsy the tail of the pancreas was replaced by an indurated, lobulated, gray-white neoplasm (Fig. 6-25) whose histological pattern was obscurely glandular, with a cell population exhibiting bizarre nuclear aberrations and gigantism (Fig. 6-26).

A 65-year-old male presented with abdominal pain and a cystic enlargement of the pancreatic body, which was probed by a fine, flexible spinal needle under CAT scan guidance (Fig. 6-27). The aspirate retrieved glandular cells of variable nuclear character with prominent, often multiple nucleoli, and pale cytoplasm arranged in a rosette around a central luminal space (Fig.

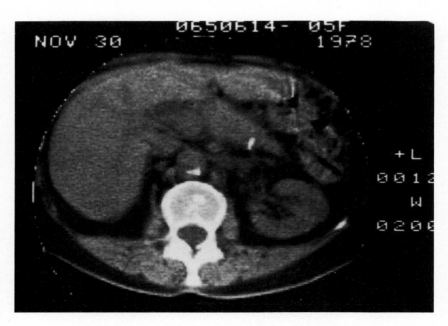

Fig. 6-22. CAT scan demonstrating enlarged pancreas with tip of needle localized to the pancreatic tail.

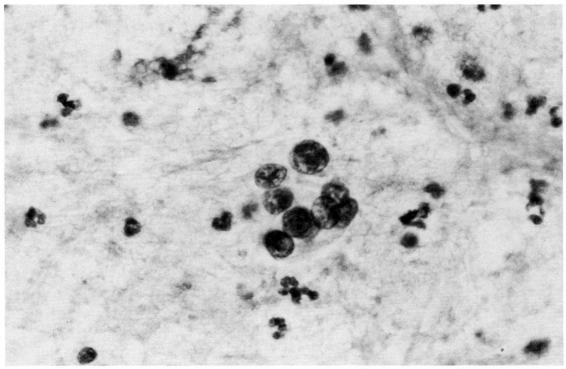

Fig. 6-23. Needle aspirate, Papanicolaou's stain, 800×, adenocarcinoma of pancreas.

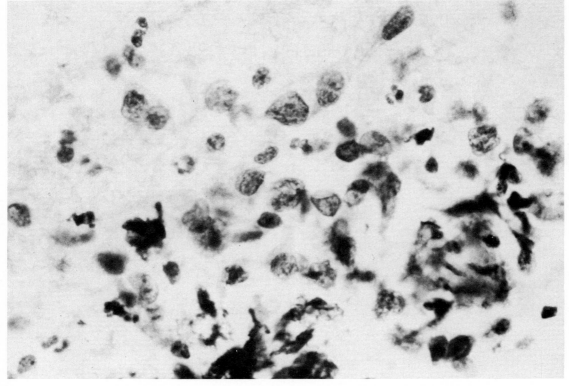

Fig. 6-24. Needle aspirate, Papanicolaou's stain, 800×, adenocarcinoma of pancreas.

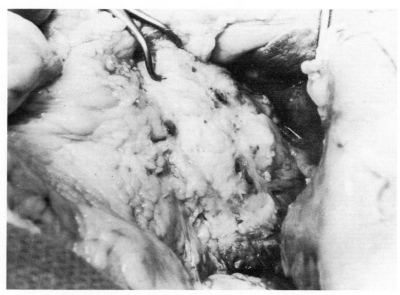

Fig. 6-25. Pancreatic mass at autopsy (stomach is deflected anteriorly).

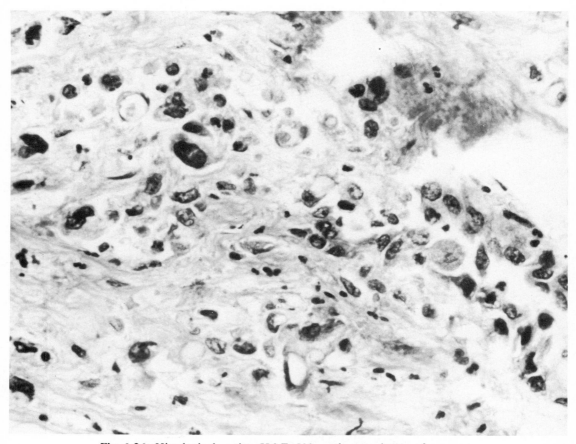

Fig. 6-26. Histological section, H & E, 500×, adenocarcinoma of pancreas.

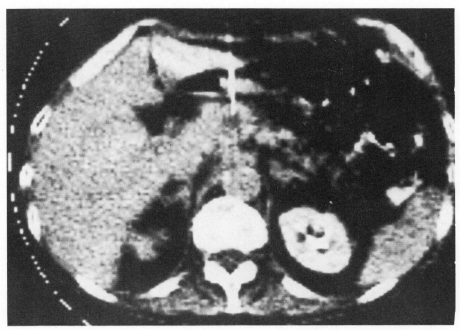

Fig. 6-27. CAT scan demonstrating needle in situ within a mass involving the body of the pancreas.

6-28). A diagnosis of adenocarcinoma of the pancreas was established. The patient was subsequently explored for obstruction and a biopsy of the omentum revealed metastatic adenocarcinoma (Fig. 6-29), providing indirect histological correlation with the aspirate.

A 74-year-old male was hospitalized for management of vomiting and diarrhea, which commenced after a syncopal episode during which he sustained head trauma. The hospital course was punctuated by upper gastrointestinal hemorrhage, pneumonia, acute renal failure, and symptoms suggesting leakage from a known abdominal aortic aneurysm. CAT scan evaluation of the abdomen disclosed a pancreatic mass that was investigated by fine needle aspiration (Fig. 6-30). The position of the needle in the enlarged pancreatic image is accentuated in the subtraction study (Fig. 6-31). The aspirated material consisted of fibrinopurulent exudate, necrotic debris, cellular detritus, and degenerated epithelium with globules suggesting lipid (Figs. 6-32, 6-33). A diagnosis of pancreatitis or pancreatic abscess was offered. The patient died on the 36th hospital day and was referred for necropsy examination. The entire pancreas was replaced by necrotic debris and fibrinopurulent

exudate, and liquefactive necrosis with saponification involved adjacent peripancreatic adipose tissue and omentum. The inflammatory process was concluded with sepsis and vascular collapse. Sections of the pancreas revealed coagulative and liquefactive necrosis with residues of lobular images (Fig. 6-34).

An 80-year-old male was evaluated by CAT examination of the abdomen because of a mass that was localized to the retroperitoneum adjacent to the left kidney near the splenic tail. A needle was directed into the lesion (Fig. 6-35) and large, dissociated polyhedral cells were extracted. The cytoplasm appeared distinct, vacuolated, clear, or granular. Oval nuclei were rather bland except for nucleolar prominence and coarse chromatin distribution (Fig. 6-36). Mucin stains were negative. The aspirate was postulated to represent an adenocarcinoma, more likely of renal cell than pancreatic origin. Confirmation was not obtained and the patient was lost to histopathological follow-up.

A 60-year-old male presented with a pelvic mass several months subsequent to cystectomy for transitional cell carcinoma of the bladder with squamoid differentiation. A CAT-scan of the pelvis demonstrated a conspicuous left retro-

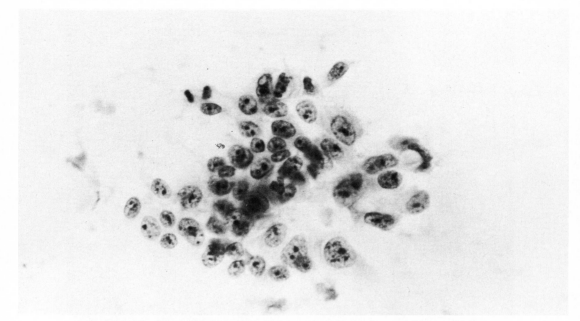

Fig. 6-28. Needle aspirate, Papanicolaou's stain, 625×, adenocarcinoma of pancreas.

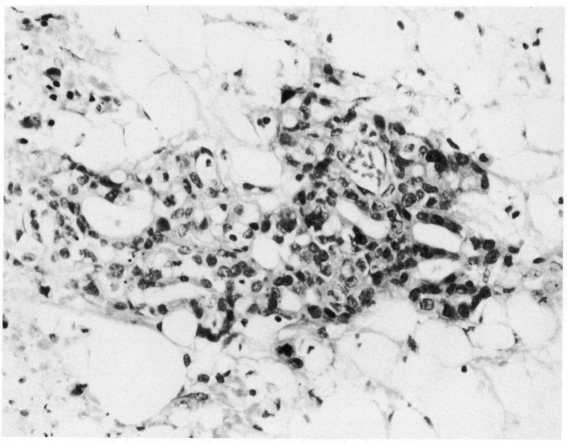

Fig. 6-29. Histological section, H&E, 400×, metastatic adenocarcinoma in omentum.

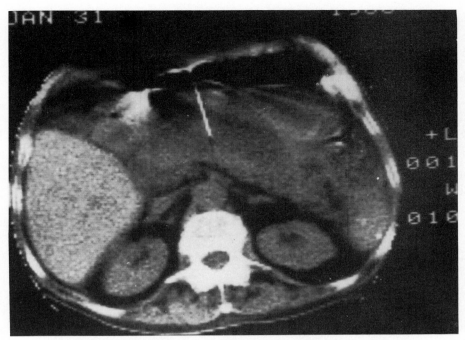

Fig. 6-30. CAT scan demonstrating enlarged pancreas with needle in target.

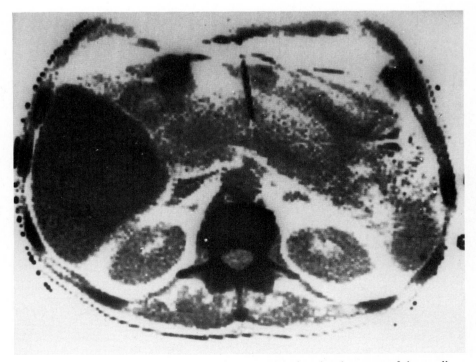

Fig. 6-31. CAT scan, subtraction technique accentuating the placement of the needle.

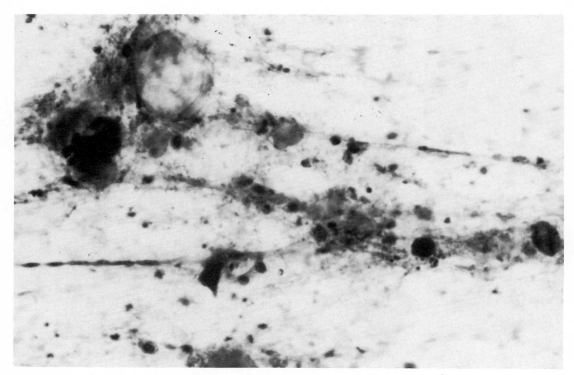

Fig. 6-32. Needle aspirate, Papanicolaou's stain, 400×, cellular detritus, necrotic debris, and lipid globules.

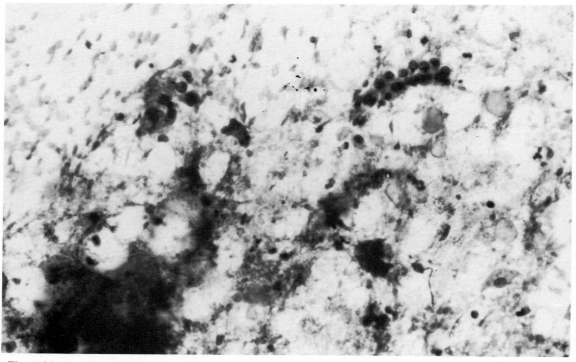

Fig. 6-33. Needle aspirate, Papanicolaou's stain, 400×, degenerated epithelial cells, necrotic debris, cellular detritus, and lipid globules.

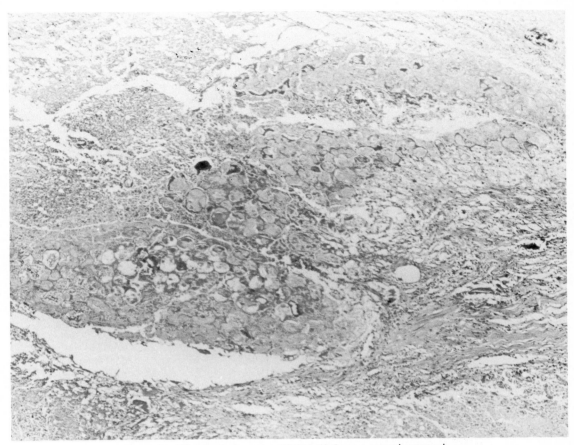

Fig. 6-34. Histological section, H&E, 62.5×, pancreatic necrosis.

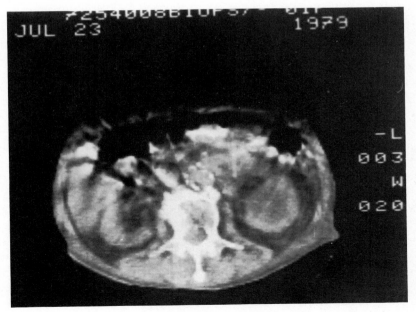

Fig. 6-35. CT scan demonstrating position of needle in left retroperitoneal mass.

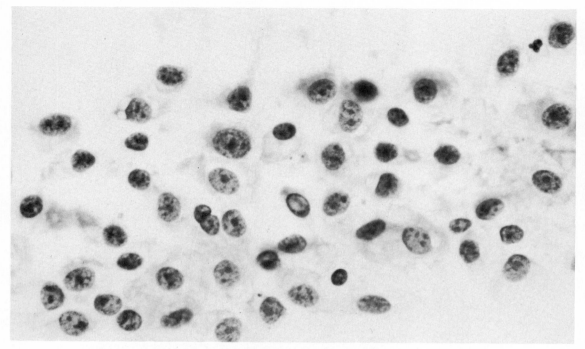

Fig. 6-36. Needle aspirate, Papanicolaou's stain, 625×, possible renal cell carcinoma.

iliac mass that was accessible to the directed needle (Fig. 6-37). Clusters of cells with nuclei of variable size and chromasia were condensed in pseudopapillary clusters without regard for orientation (Fig. 6-38). Pearl formations suggested a capability for squamoid differentiation. The cells corresponded to the epithelium of the primary bladder neoplasm, which deeply invaded smooth muscle (Fig. 6-39).

A 60-year-old male with antecedent history of transitional cell carcinoma of the bladder presented with a left suprarenal mass that was referred for CAT scan directed fine needle aspiration (Fig. 6-40). The cells were arranged in papillary aggregates and exhibited subtle variations in shape with modest anisokaryosis (Fig. 6-41). Nucleoli were exaggerated within the vesicular nucleoplasm. Cytoplasm appeared indistinct. The cells were considered to represent metastases from the previous transitional cell carcinoma, which was composed of similar cells arranged in papillary upheaval on delicate, vascularized connective tissue stalks (Fig. 6-42).

A 62-year-old male presented with fever and abdominal pain. An abdominal CAT scan localized a large right retroperitoneal mass that was

approached from a posterior puncture under CAT guidance (Fig. 6-43). The aspirate consisted exclusively of fibrinopurulent exudate (Fig. 6-44). A second pass was done for additional tissue to inoculate culture media and *Salmonella choleraesuis* was isolated in essentially pure culture. After decompression and antibiotic therapy, the patient was explored for evacuation and resection of a residual abscess wall, fortified by skeletal muscle in transition with granulation tissue and fibrinopurulent exudate (Fig. 6-45). No tumor was identified.

A 73-year-old male presented with a right upper quadrant mass localized to the retroperitoneum by CAT. Directed needle penetration through a posterior approach (Fig. 6-46) permitted the isolation of a monomorphous population of round cells with minimal cytoplasm, nuclear probosci, indentations, visible nucleoli, and coarse chromatin particles (Fig. 6-47). A diagnosis of lymphoma, suggesting poorly differentiated lymphocytic type was suggested and confirmed by retroperitoneal biopsies at laparotomy. Sheets of monomorphous cells with cleftular indentations, extensions of the nuclear envelopes, and coarse hyperchromasia (Fig.

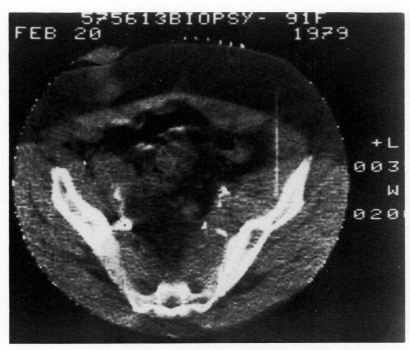

Fig. 6-37. CT scan demonstrating placement of needle in left retroiliac mass.

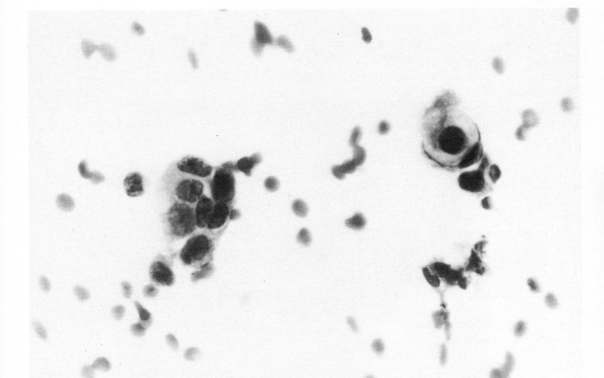

Fig. 6-38. Needle aspirate, Papanicolaou's stain, 800×, metastatic transitional cell carcinoma with squamoid features.

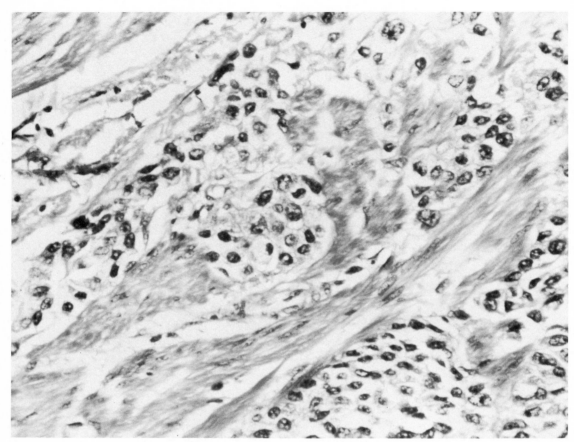

Fig. 6-39. Histological section, H&E, primary transitional cell carcinoma of bladder involving smooth muscle (cystectomy specimen).

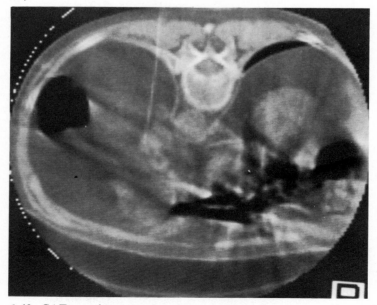

Fig. 6-40. CAT scan demonstrating placement of needle in left suprarenal mass.

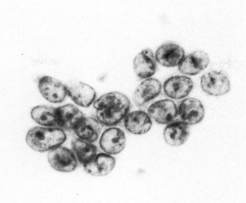

Fig. 6-41. Needle aspirate, Papanicolaou's stain, 800×, papillary transitional cell carcinoma.

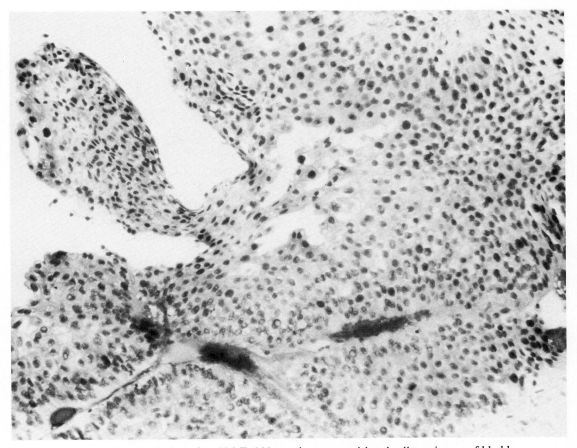

Fig. 6-42. Histological section, H&E, 200×, primary transitional cell carcinoma of bladder.

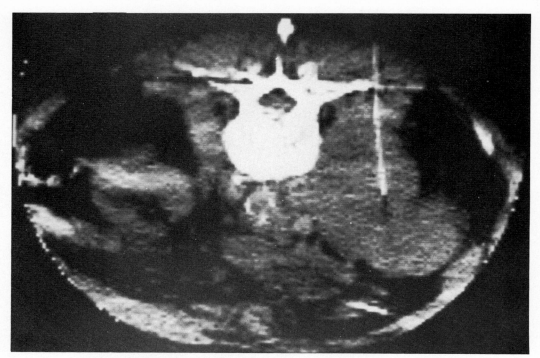

Fig. 6-43. CAT scan demonstrating needle in right retroperitoneal mass.

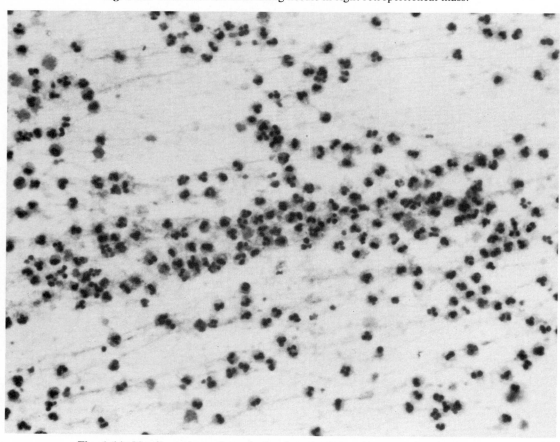

Fig. 6-44. Needle aspirate, Papanicolaou's stain, 500×, fibrinopurulent exudate.

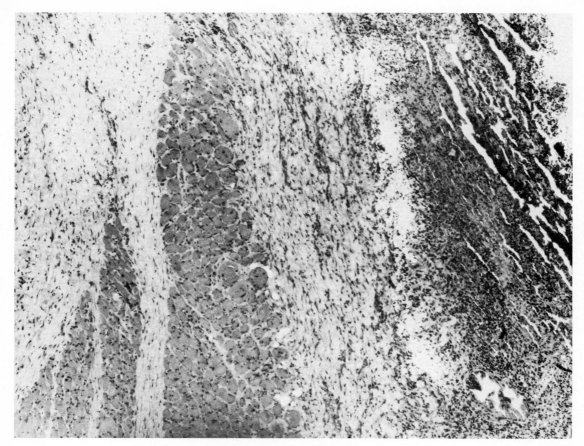

Fig. 6-45. Histological section, H&E, 80×, abscess wall.

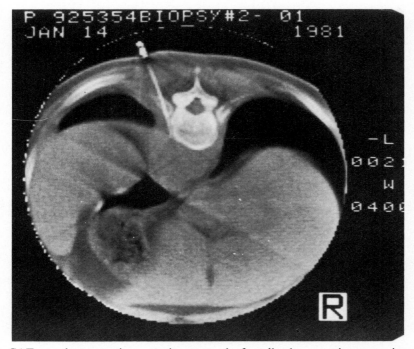

Fig. 6-46. CAT scan demonstrating posterior approach of needle placement in retroperitoneal mass.

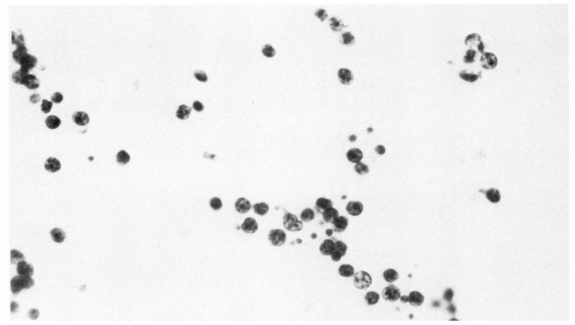

Fig. 6-47. Needle aspirate, Papanicolaou's stain, 625×, malignant lymphoma.

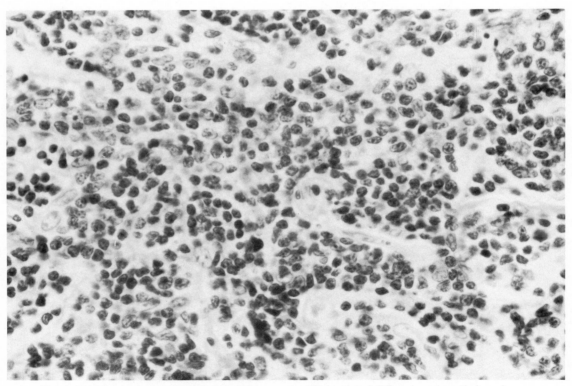

Fig. 6-48. Histological section, H&E, 800×, poorly differentiated diffuse lymphocytic lymphoma.

6-48) were considered diagnostic of poorly differentiated, diffuse lymphocytic lymphoma. Chemotherapy was initiated but the patient deteriorated with fever, leukocytosis, and thrombocytopenia. At the postmortem examination, tumor extended from its origin in the retroperitoneum at the porta hepatis to displace the transverse colon anteriorly and the small bowel inferiorly, with direct involvement of colonic wall, duodenum, pancreas, and adrenals. Lymph node conglomerates were universally replaced by tumor. Although needle aspiration cannot provide classification of the type of lymphoma or predict its organizational status (diffuse or nodular), the cytology of the proliferating element may be characterized sufficiently to predict malignant lymphoma and perhaps provoke further biopsy for tissue analysis.

Two years following excision of a villous adenoma of the rectum, a 50-year-old woman was evaluated for a pelvic mass in the retrorectal tissues. A CAT scan assisted fine needle aspirate was performed through a posterior (gluteal) approach (Fig. 6-49). Rare clusters of malignant glandular cells in trabecular alignment were diagnostic for adenocarcinoma (Fig. 6-50). It

was suggested that the initial villous adenoma may have contained an occult focus of carcinoma that recurred with time. Conventional biopsy was deferred.

INVESTIGATION OF PARENCHYMAL LESIONS OF LIVER

Fine needle aspiration of the liver can obtain comprehensive information concerning the occurrence of acute hepatitis, cirrhosis, steatosis, hemosiderosis, and metabolic inborn errors in addition to confirming primary or secondary malignant disease.[38] Satisfactory specimens for cytological analysis can be achieved in as many as 99% of biopsies without threat of serious complications or mortality. Lundquist reported no occurrence of death, and only one serious complication, an intrahepatic hematoma that required surgical evacuation, in 2611 biopsies constituting his experience. Analysis of 1748 aspiration biopsies provided a cytological diagnosis of cancer in 57 instances. There were no false positives, but 15 false negatives were recorded. Arteriography and scintigraphy were

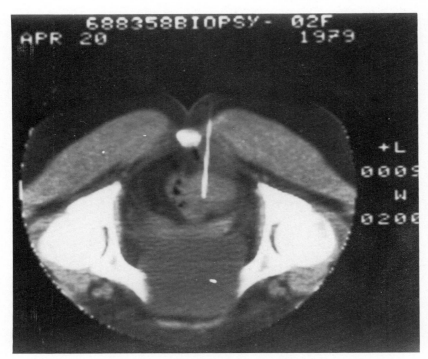

Fig. 6-49. CAT scan demonstrating transgluteal posterior approach. The needle is in a retrorectal mass.

occasionally utilized but the advantage of CAT scan directed techniques was unavailable.

We have extensively utilized CAT to direct the thin needle into intrahepatic targets to insure a profitable cellular harvest; guided placement of the needle has succeeded in obtaining diagnostic material when conventional thick-bore biopsy needles used for blind sampling of the hepatic parenchyma have failed. There have been no clinically significant complications or false positive results. Figure 6-51 demonstrates the position of the needle probe in an area of lucency within the liver of a 50-year-old male with antecedent history of squamous cell carcinoma of the lung. The needle aspirate harvested cells in cohesive mosaic nests with communal affinity assured by the presence of intercellular adhesive filaments (Fig. 6-52). The hyperchromatic nuclei with coarse chromatin and tendency to spindling contributed additional evidence for a squamous character. A diagnosis of metastatic squamous cell carcinoma was established, and no further attempt was made to obtain tissue. Chemotherapy was initiated based on the cell-type projected by the cytological appearance. A 78-year-old male with cough, weight loss, and a left hilar mass (Fig. 6-53) was evaluated by CAT scan of the abdomen for liver function abnormalities in association with hepatomegaly. Multiple lucencies were identified within the enlarged liver (Fig. 6-54) and it was elected to investigate presumed hepatic metastases with aspiration biopsy. The cellular harvest consisted of small round or spindle cells with hyperchromatic nuclei, minimal cytoplasm and molding (Fig. 6-55), diagnostic of metastatic undifferentiated carcinoma, oat cell type. A conventional thick bore parenchymal biopsy needle was utilized to obtain tissue (Fig. 6-56) by blind puncture, but the tumor was inadvertently missed. Directed biopsy with cytological preparation can offer a more scientific approach to cellular acquisition.

A 76-year-old-woman with antecedent history of modified radical mastectomy for infiltrating duct cell carcinoma presented with abnormal liver chemistries and a defect in the liver demonstrated by CAT (Fig. 6-57). The needle was

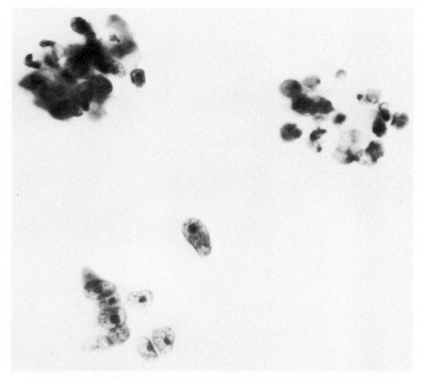

Fig. 6-50. Needle aspirate, Papanicolaou's stain, 800×, adenocarcinoma.

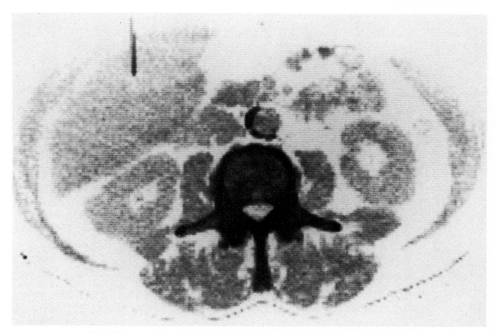

Fig. 6-51. CAT scan demonstrating needle within hepatic lesion.

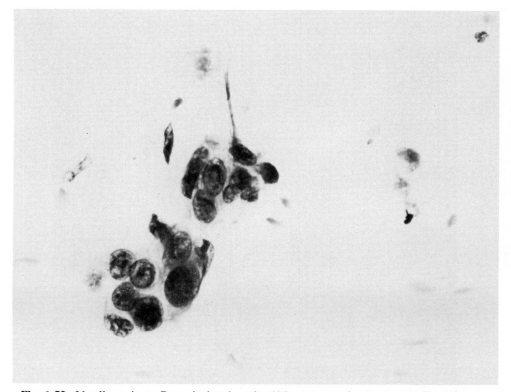

Fig. 6-52. Needle aspirate, Papanicolaou's stain, 625×, metastatic squamous cell carcinoma.

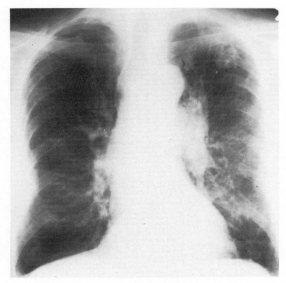

Fig. 6-53. Chest x-ray, AP projection demonstrating left hilar mass.

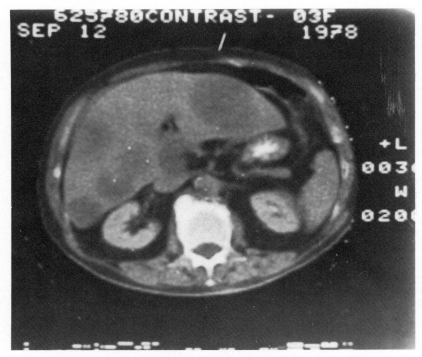

Fig. 6-54. CAT scan demonstrating multiple lucencies in liver.

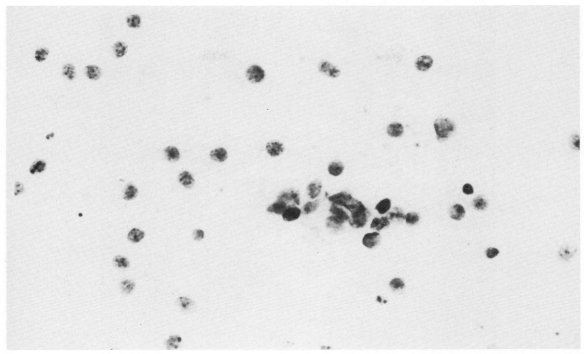

Fig. 6-55. Needle aspirate, Papanicolaou's stain, 625×, metastatic small cell undifferentiated carcinoma, oat cell type.

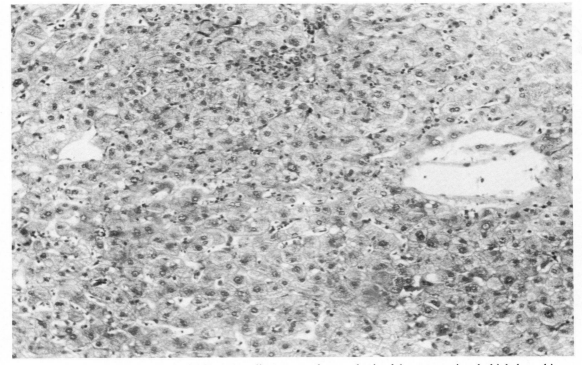

Fig. 6-56. Histological section, H&E, 160×, liver parenchyma obtained by conventional thick bore biopsy needle. No tumor identified.

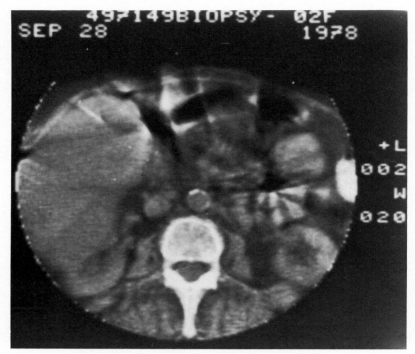

Fig. 6-57. CAT scan demonstrating placement of needle within an hepatic mass.

inserted in the lesion under CAT guidance and epithelial cells arranged in acini (Fig. 6-58) were retrieved. The columnar cells exhibited nuclear variations in size, chromatin texture, and contour. A diagnosis of metastatic breast carci-

Fig. 6-58. Needle aspirate, Papanicolaou's stain, 625×, metastatic adenocarcinoma consistent with origin from breast primary.

noma was confirmed by subsequent conventional needle biopsy requested by a skeptical oncologist. The histological appearance verified metastatic epithelial cells arranged in trabecular cords and abortive acini (Fig. 6-59).

A 68-year old woman presented with elevations of the alkaline phosphatase and gamma glutamyl transpeptidase. A liver scan revealed radionuclide defects suggesting metastatic disease. A radical mastectomy had been performed 10 years earlier for duct cell carcinoma of the breast. A conventional liver biopsy performed blindly showed recent perivenular hepatocellular necrosis but no tumor was identified. She was therefore considered a candidate for CAT directed fine needle aspiration and the needle was positioned in a selected target (Fig. 6-60). The cellular material was scarce but consisted of large columnar cells with nuclei of variable size, prominent nucleoli, and a suggestively glandular configuration (Fig. 6-61). Chemotherapy was administered on the presumptive evidence that the tumor was consistent with origin from the ancient primary.

The diagnosis of lymphoma can be projected from the cytological preparation but classifica-

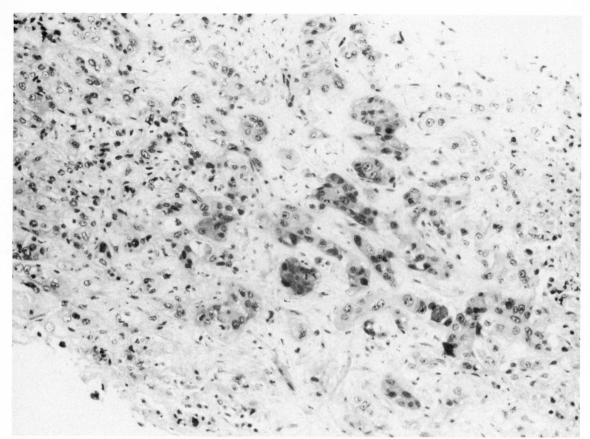

Fig. 6-59. Histological section, H&E, 200×, conventional thick bore biopsy needle, metastatic adenocarcinoma consistent with origin from breast primary.

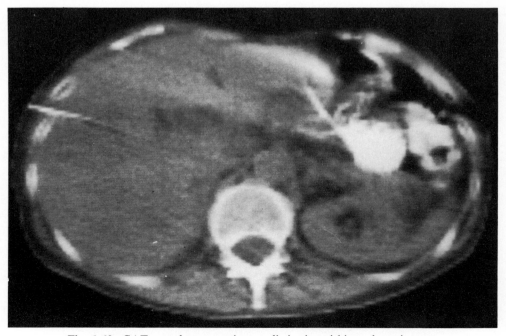

Fig. 6-60. CAT scan demonstrating needle in situ within an hepatic mass.

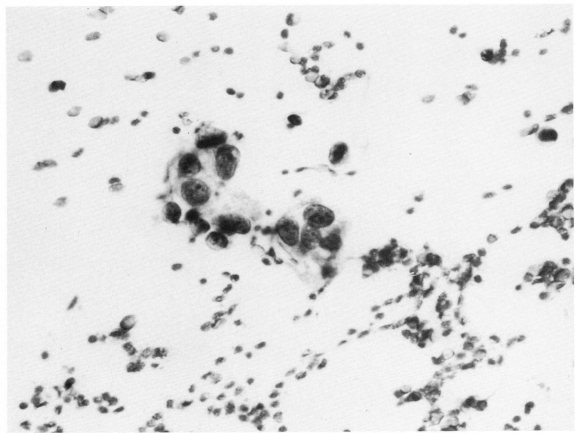

Fig. 6-61. Needle aspirate, Papanicolaou's stain, 500×, metastatic adenocarcinoma consistent with origin from breast primary.

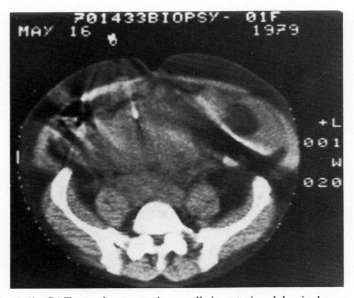

Fig. 6-62. CAT scan demonstrating needle in anterior abdominal mass.

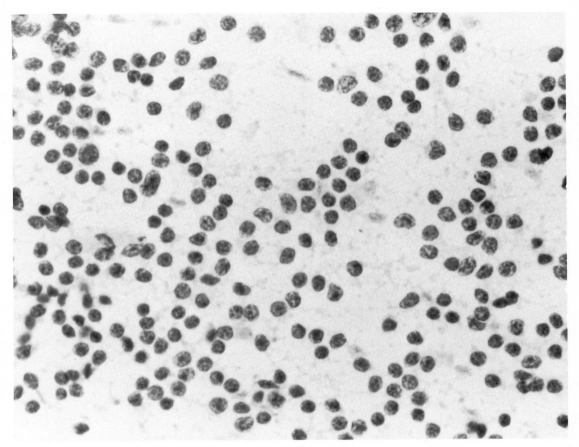

Fig. 6-63. Needle aspirate, Papanicolaou's stain, 625×, malignant lymphoma.

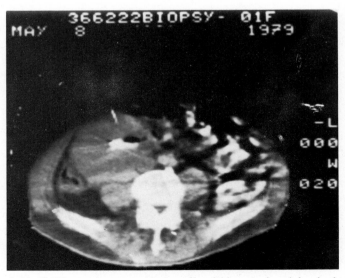

Fig. 6-64. CAT scan demonstrating needle within anterior abdominal mass.

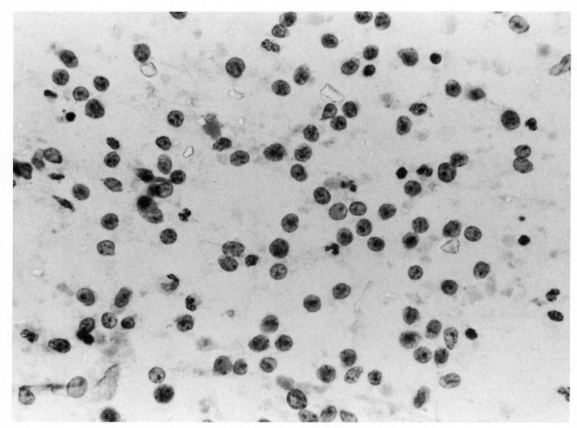

Fig. 6-65. Needle aspirate, Papanicolaou's stain, 625×, malignant lymphoma.

tion according to the criteria of Lukes or Rappaport, or prediction about the architectural arrangement of the lymphoma in solid tissue (nodular versus diffuse) may be quite inaccurate and the limitations of aspiration cytology in the investigation of malignant lymphoma must be stressed. The one possible exception is in recognition of Hodgkin's disease because the characteristic Reed-Sternberg cell is unique, but not specific to lymphoma. A 68-year-old male with lymphadenopathy, hepatomegaly, and a palpable abdominal mass was evaluated by CAT directed biopsy of the anterior mass, presumptively in contiguity with liver (Fig. 6-62). The cells consisted of round or angular lymphocytes with coarse chromatin dispersion, slight variability in size, and vehement tendency for dissociation and isolated disportation (Fig. 6-63). Malignant lymphoma was diagnosed but no tissue follow-up was available for further classification. Chemotherapy was initiated. A 73-year-old male with clinical evidence for a tumor involving the liver was investigated by aspiration biopsy under CAT guidance (Fig. 6-64). The cells resembled large lymphocytes of uniform size with slightly variable nuclear contours, prominent nucleoli, and stippled chromatin arranged without regard for cohesion (Fig. 6-65). A diagnosis of poorly differentiated lymphocytic lymphoma was proposed and retroperitoneal biopsies were obtained at laparotomy. The tumor consisted of comparable cells arranged in arbitrary diffuse sheets (Fig. 6-66) constituting the architecture of a 20-cm mass. Combined systemic chemotherapy was initiated but the patient died with extensive intra-abdominal dissemination and lymph node conglomeration.

We have not attempted to utilize the technique for a "medical" biopsy to investigate the presence of hepatitis, iron, or enzymes, but certainly the versatility of the approach would support creative utilization for inspecting the liver at a cellular threshold.

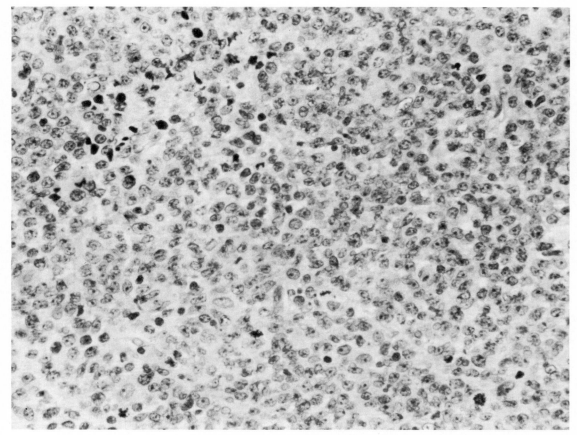

Fig. 6-66. Histological section, H&E, 500×, poorly differentiated, diffuse lymphocytic lymphoma.

REFERENCES

1. Haaga, J. R., and Alfidi, R. J.: Precise biopsy localization by computed tomography. *Radiology* **118:** 603–607, 1976.
2. Hounsfield, G. N.: Computerized transverse axial scanning (tomography), part I. Description of system. *Br J Radiol* **46:** 1016–1022, 1973.
3. Kreel, L.: Computerized tomography using the EMI general purpose scanner. *Br J Radiol* **50**(589): 2–24, 1977.
4. Alfidi, R. J., and Haaga, J. R.: Computed body tomography. *Radiol Clin North Am* **14**(3): 563–570, 1976.
5. Wittenberg, J., and Ferrucci, J. T., Jr.: Computed body tomography. *Gastroenterology* **74:** 287, 1978.
6. Gado, M. H., Phelps, M. D., and Colman, R. E.: An extravascular component of contrast enhancement in cranial computed tomography (parts I and II). *Radiology* **117:** 589–597, 1975.
7. Moss, A. A., Kressel, H. Y., Korobkin, M., Goldberg, H. I., Rohlfing, B. M., and Brasch, R. C.: The effect of gastrografin and glucagon on CT scanning of the pancreas: A blind clinical trial. *Radiology* **126**(3): 711–714, 1978.
8. Robbins, A. H., Pugatch, R. D., Gerzof, S. G., Faling, L. J., Johnson, W. C., and Sewell, D. H.: Observations on medical efficiency of computed tomography of chest and abdomen. *Am J R* **131:** 15, 1978.
9. Kressel, H. Y., Callen, P. W., Montagne, J. P., Korobkin, M., Goldberg, H. I., Moss, A. A., Arger, P. H., and Margulis, A. R.: Computed tomographic evaluation of disorders affecting the alimentary tract. *Radiology* **129:** 451–455, 1978.
10. Kreel, L. M., Haertel, M., and Katz, D.: Computed tomography of the normal pancreas. *J Comput Assist Tomogr* **1**(3): 290–299, 1977.
11. Husband, J. E., and Kreel, L.: Computerized tomography in the localization of abdominal malignancy. *J R Soc Med* **71**(1): 35–38, 1978.
12. Ferrucci, J. T. Jr.: Diagnosis of abdominal malignancy by fine needle aspiration. *Am J R* **134:** 323–330, 1980.
13. Holm, H. H., Pedersen, J. F., Kristensen, J. K., Rasmussen, S., Hancke, S., and Jensen, F. Ultrasonically-guided percutaneous puncture. *Radiol Clin North Am* **13:** 493–503, 1975.
14. Hancke, S., Holm, H. H., and Koch, F.: Ultrasonically-guided percutaneous fine needle biopsy of the pancreas. *Surg, Gynecol Obstet* **140:** 361–364, 1975.
15. Haaga, J. R., Reech, N. E., Havrilla, T. R., and Alfidi, R.: Interventional CT scanning. *Radiol Clin North Am* **15:** 449–456, 1977.
16. Pereiras, R. V., Meurs, A., and Kinhardt, B.: Fluoroscopically-guided thin needle aspiration biopsy of the abdomen and retroperitoneum. *Am J R* **131:** 197–202, 1978.

17. Goldstein, H. M., Zornoza, J., and Wallace, S.: Percutaneous fine needle aspiration biopsy of pancreatic and other abdominal masses. *Radiology* **123**: 319–322, 1977.

18. Gothlin, J. H.: Post-lymphographic percutaneous fine needle biopsy of lymph nodes guided by fluoroscopy. *Radiology* **120**: 205–207, 1977.

19. Zornoza, J., Jonsson, K., Wallace, S., and Lukeman, J.: Fine needle aspiration biopsy of retroperitoneal lymph nodes and abdominal masses: An updated report. *Radiology* **125**: 87–88, 1977.

20. Burcharth, F., and Rasmussen, S. N.: Localization of the porta hepatis by ultrasonic scanning prior to percutaneous transhepatic portography. *Br J Radiol* **47**: 598–602, 1974.

21. Ho, C. S., McLaughlin, M. J., McHattie, J. D., and Tao, L.: Percutaneous fine needle aspiration biopsy of the pancreas following endoscopic retrograde cholangiopancreatopgraphy. *Radiology* **125**: 351–353, 1977.

22. Tylen, U., Arnesgo, B., Lundberg, L. G., and Lunderquist, A.: Percutaneous biopsy of carcinoma of the pancreas guided by angiography. *Surg, Gynecol Obstet* **142**: 737–739, 1976.

23. Ferrucci, J. T., and Wittenberg, J.: CT biopsy of abdominal tumors: Aids for lesion localization. *Radiology* **129**: 739–744, 1978.

24. Goldberg, B. B., and Pollack, H. M.: Ultrasonic aspiration-biopsy transducer. *Radiology* **108**: 667–671, 1973.

25. Haaga, J. R., and Reech, N. E.: *Computed Tomography of Abdominal Abnormalities. CT-guided Needle Procedures and Current Status and Future Direction.* C. V. Mosby, St. Louis, 1978.

26. Ferrucci, J. T. Jr., Wittenberg, J., and Sarno, R. A.: Fine needle transhepatic cholangiography: A new approach to obstructive jaundice. *Am J R* **127**: 403–407, 1976.

27. Ferrucci, J. T. Jr., Wittenberg, J., Margolies, M. N., and Carey, R. W.: Malignant seeding of needle tract after thin needle aspiration biopsy: A previously unrecorded complication. *Radiology* **130**: 345–346, 1979.

28. Engzell, U., Esposti, P. L., Rubio, C., Sigurdson, A., and Zajicek, J.: Investigation in tumors spread in connection with aspiration biopsy. *Acta Radiol Oncol Radiat Phys Biol* **10**: 385–388, 1971.

29. Sinner, W. N., and Zajicek, J.: Implantation metastasis after percutaneous transthoracic needle aspiration biopsy. *Acta Radiol Oncol Radiol Phys Biol* **17**: 473–480, 1976.

30. Crele, G., and Hayard, J. B.: Classification of thyroiditis with special reference to the use of needle biopsy. *J Clin Endocrinol Metab* **11**: 1123–1127, 1951.

31. Clark, B. G., Leadbetter, W. F., and Campbell, J. S.: Implantation of cancer of the prostate in site of perineal needle biopsy: Report of a case. *J Urol* **70**: 937–939, 1953.

32. Wolinsky, H., and Lischner, M. A.: Needle tract implantation after percutaneous lung biopsy. *Ann Intern Med* **71**: 349–362, 1969.

33. Berg, J. W., and Robbins, G. F.: A late look at the safety of aspiration biopsy. *Cancer* **15**: 826–827, 1962.

34. Robbins, G. F., Brothers, J. H. Eberhart, W. F., and Quan, S.: Is aspiration biopsy of breast cancer dangerous to the patient? *Cancer* **7**: 774–778, 1954.

35. VonSchreeb, T., Arner, O., Skovsted, G., and Wilkstad, N.: Renal adenocarcinoma. Is there a risk of spreading tumor cells in diagnostic puncture. *Scand J Urol Nephrol* **1**: 270–276, 1967.

36. Kline, T. S., Abramson, J., Goldstein, F., and Neal, H. S.: Needle aspiration biopsy of the pancreas at laparotomy. *Am J Gastroenterol* **68**: 30–33, 1977.

37. McLoughlin, M. J.: Fine needle aspiration biopsy of malignant lesions in and around the pancreas. *Cancer* **41**: 2413–2419, 1978.

38. Lundquist, A.: Fine needle aspiration biopsy of the liver: Applications in clinical diagnosis and investigation. *Acta Med Scand (Suppl)* **520**: 1–28, 1971.

The Direct-Visualization Biopsy: Surface Aspirates

The occurrence of a visible mass that distorts appearance, or by its strategic location interferes with usual function, provokes concern that challenges the patient's comfort and eventuates in his seeking medical advice. A surface mass constitutes an essential indication for biopsy, and thin needle aspiration is the vehicle for conservative, precise intervention and a rapid diagnosis. The subcutaneous geography relieves the cytopathologist of the necessity for ancillary radiographic devices for localization and targeting. The implements are fundamental, the approach sophisticated, and the results readily obtained and accurate. This chapter is intended to stimulate flirtation with the permutations of cellular experience that may derive from the aspiration of an intriguing soft tissue mass, lymph node, or parotid swelling, to excite the reader into exploration, reconnaissance of the literature, and a sense of awareness to investigate the visible palpable surface lesion. The definitive work in the cytopathology of sarcomas already exists[1] and may serve to guide a redefinition of terms in the transition from exfoliative studies to needle acquisition. In addition, there will be brief reference to examination of bone lesions.

SOFT TISSUE NODULES

The experience of fine needle aspiration cytology applied to soft tissue lesions, particularly sarcomas, is limited despite the indications. The justifications reside in the concepts that radical excision of a soft tissue sarcoma is more readily achieved when the tumor has not been previously exposed for biopsy[2] and that incisional biopsy may seed the wound when definitive resection does not follow. It is necessary to differentiate between a metastatic carcinoma and a primary sarcoma or lymphoma cutis. Verification of a metastatic deposit may circumvent alternative, often expensive, invasive procedures or radiographic staging technics. Disclosure is mandatory when an inflammatory or traumatic-reparative lesion arises in mimicry of a malignant process.

The sporadic reports speak of confidence and promise. Akerman[2] obtained sufficient material for diagnosis in 92% of the 178 patients with soft tissue lesions diagnosed by fine needle aspiration with conventional technique. The cytological diagnosis was accurate in 88% of the malignant and 95% of the benign cases. Kline's[3] group achieved an accuracy of 95% of their 88 malignant neoplasms, but their analysis included lymph node punctures, which may bias their statistics. Frable[9] correctly characterized 52 soft masses as benign or malignant. Although he admitted that specific classification of a sarcoma may be difficult by this method, substantiation of a tumor as a sarcoma was quite reasonably achieved, and he correctly identified a liposarcoma and chordoma. Hajdu and Melamed[11] examined 43 soft tissue lesions by aspiration and correctly identified cancer in all instances.

There are numerous factors that inflict obstacles to accurate diagnosis of soft tissue lesions. A preponderantly fibrous matrix may tenaciously retain cells, in a posture of reluctant dissociation.

The fibroblasts of repair may be visibly atypical, often ominous, with a proliferative frenzy that compares to cells sampled from aggressive fibromatoses or recapitulated in neurinomas. A fibroblastic synovial sarcoma may resemble a benign neurogenic tumor.[2] Tumors with cystic or necrotic centers encourage desquamation to the internal liquid milieu where degeneration proceeds without restriction or recompense. The reports of sampling soft tissue masses implicitly state that metastatic epithelial malignancies are easier to recognize with assurance, and there may be a tendency to quantitate this more familiar entity. In the Memorial Hospital study,[11] 33 of the 43 aspirated soft tissue lesions were metastatic (33% epidermoid and 56% adenocarcinoma). At the Medical College of Virginia[9] 22 of the 28 malignant soft tissue masses were metastatic carcinomas, predominantly from breast and lung.

The technique may be applied with impunity in terms of complications. There is no significant risk of tumor implantation along the needle tract,[2,3] clinically significant hemorrhage, or infection.

A few examples from our files may indicate the quality and diversity of the cellular harvest from soft tissue masses to support our contention of its applicability.

A 76-year-old male presented with a subcutaneous swelling in the region of his right deltoid muscle and a needle aspirate was prepared according to conventional technique. The pleomorphic cellular population was dominated by polyhedral and spindle cells (Fig. 7-1) singly disported in a milieu of inflammation and cellular detritus. The nuclei appeared enlarged, irregular, hyperchromatic, and often duplicate, particularly in cells with tapered cytoplasm containing fibrillations but no definitive actinomyosin filaments. A striking eosinophilia, often with an homogenized quality, was noted in fusiform cells. A diagnosis of myosarcoma was postulated and excisional biopsy was subse-

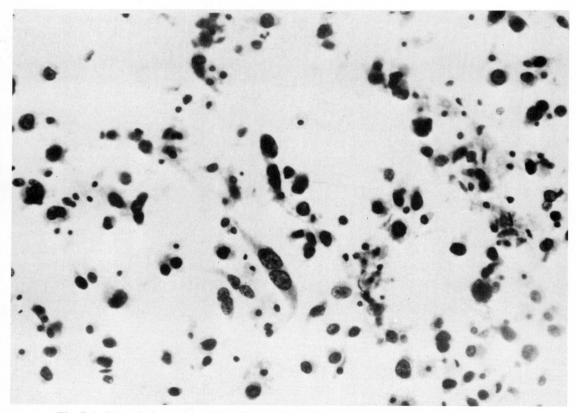

Fig. 7-1. Papanicolaou stain, 400×, fine needle aspirate, pleomorphic rhabdomyosarcoma.

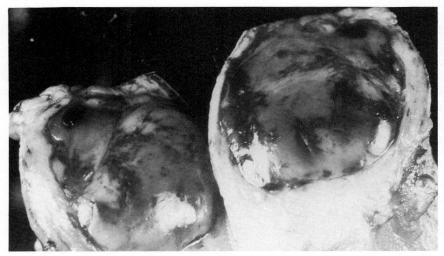

Fig. 7-2. Gross excision, rhabdomyosarcoma with variegation and hemorrhage.

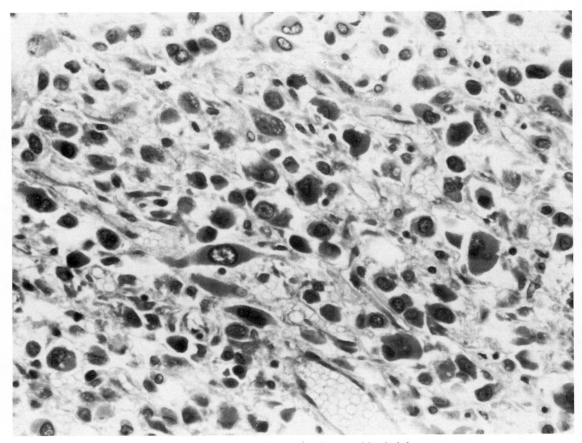

Fig. 7-3. Histologic section, H&E, 500×, pleomorphic rhabdomyosarcoma.

quently conducted. An encapsulated, variegated, fleshy, focally hemorrhagic mass was excised (Fig. 7-2). Histologic sections (Fig. 7-3) corroborated the diagnosis of myosarcoma. Polyhedral and spindled giant cells were arranged in reticulated fascicles nourished by a luxuriant capillary plexus. Broad strap cells (Fig. 7-4) gave credence to an interpretation of pleomorphic rhabdomyosarcoma, although definitive cross striations were never unequivocally demonstrated in Zenker's fixed sections.

Contrast the sarcoma pictured in Figures 7-1 to 7-4 with the appearance of binucleate giant cells from a needle aspirate of a soft tissue mass in a middle-aged woman. The nuclear margins are serrated (Fig. 7-5), chromatin is accentuated along internal folds created by membrane convolutions, and cytoplasm is abundant, and delicately vesicular. When the cells are united in congeries of four or six (Fig. 7-6), an irregular network is created in which a tendency to spindle may be subtly discerned. These cells were considered to represent derivatives from a liposarcoma, and a subsequent excisional biopsy

provided an estimate of their relationship and morphology in community organization (Fig. 7-7).

A 1.5-cm nodule in the scalp of a 73-year-old man was assessed by needle puncture and a cohesive aggregate of large, polyhedral cells with vesicular nuclei and conspicuous nucleoli was retrieved (Fig. 7-8). Chromatin was delicately dispersed around the clear zone circumscribing single or duplicate nucleoli. The abundant cytoplasm was distinctly granular but unobtrusive, with coalescence of margins into a syncytium of protoplasm reminiscent of histiocytes. Adenocarcinoma was suggested as a differential possibility, particularly because of cytoplasmic vacuolization that suggested a signet ring configuration. Multinucleated giant cells were not seen in the cytologic preparation. Sarcoma was not suspected until the excisional biopsy (Fig. 7-9) disclosed infiltration and obscuration of dermal architecture by a histiocytic lesion with occasional multinucleated histiocytes, and classification as a malignant fibrous histiocytoma was forthcoming. Our experience with aspiration of

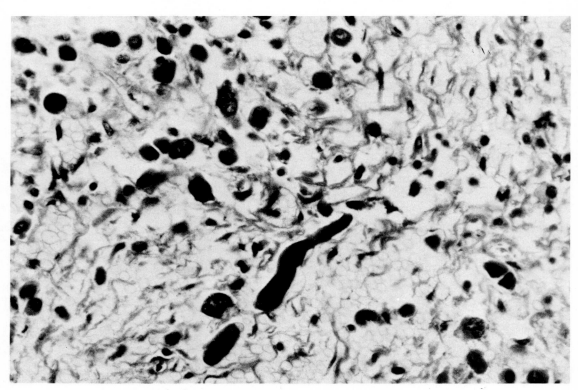

Fig. 7-4. Histologic section, H&E, 500× pleomorphic rhabdomyosarcoma.

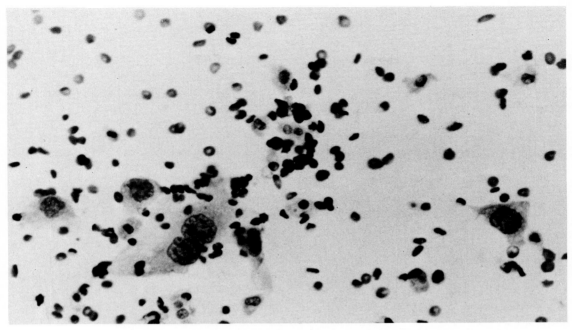

Fig. 7-5. Papanicolaou stain, 500×, fine needle aspirate, liposarcoma.

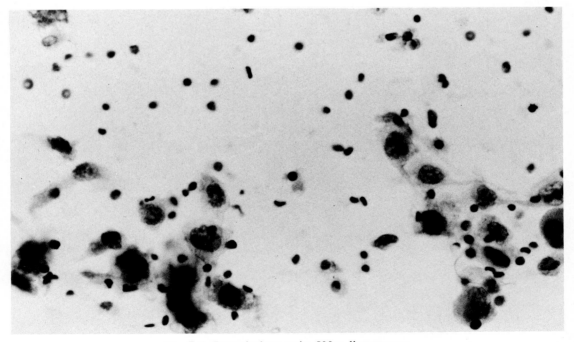

Fig. 7-6. Papanicolaou stain, 500×, liposarcoma.

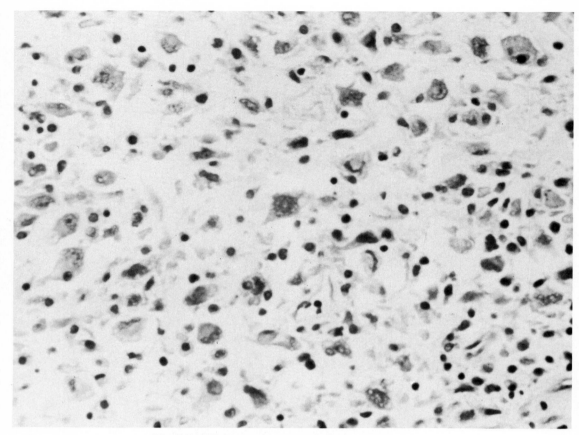

Fig. 7-7. Histologic section, H&E, 400×, liposarcoma.

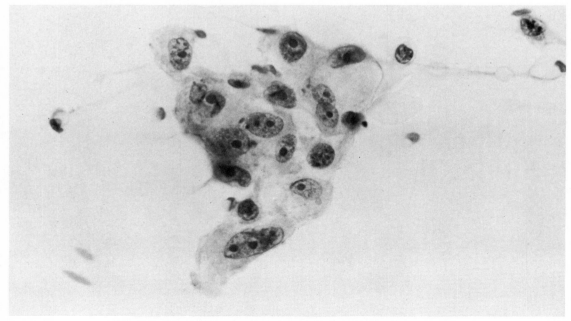

Fig. 7-8. Papanicolaou stain, 625×, malignant fibrous histiocytoma.

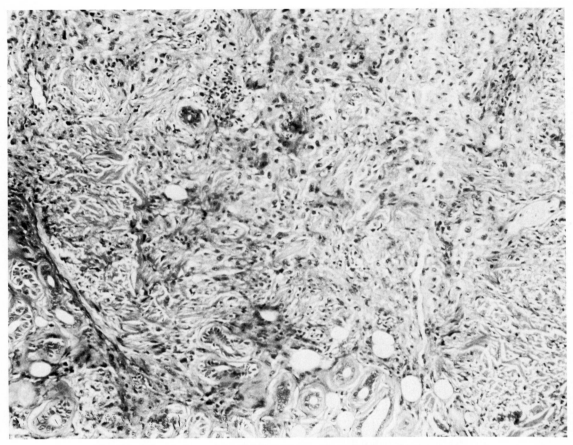

Fig. 7-9. Histologic section, H&E, 160×, malignant fibrous histiocytoma.

soft tissue swellings reflects the reported interludes with metastatic epithelial tumors. Our cases have presented with visible nodules on the back or extremities, occasionally the face. A 76-year-old male presented with a 1.5-cm protuberant induration on his left arm. The skin was slightly discolored but not ulcerated (Fig. 7-10). A needle aspirate was obtained without local anesthesia and provided a luxuriant population of small, hyperchromatic round and fusiform cells with nuclear molding, ambivalent tendency for communal affiliation and smudging (Fig. 7-11). Subsequent excisional biopsy confirmed the cytopathologist's opinion of metastatic small cell undifferentiated carcinoma from a pulmonary primary (Fig. 7-12). A bronchogenic squamous cell carcinoma was responsible for a metastatic implant in the subcutaneous interscapular area of a 66-year-old male. The aspirate (Fig. 7-13) contained keratinized spindle cells and polyhedral elements composing characteristic

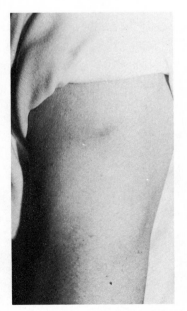

Fig. 7-10. Clinical photograph, nodule left arm, metastatic undifferentiated small cell carcinoma.

pearls in a background of necrosis, inflammation and diathesis. The tumor had evidently infarcted at the center and the liquefactive detritus was sampled by the needle which traversed the viable peripheral tissue to reach a necrotic target. Biopsy from the intact wall of the cystic implant obtained a characteristic squamous mosaic with intercellular bridges and keratinization (Fig. 7-14).

We include salivary gland enlargements in the category of soft tissue protuberances for convenience, because our material is limited, and because the presentation is often a nonlymphoid enlargement in the soft tissues of the head or neck region. Our most fascinating case is a parotid swelling of twenty years duration in an 80-year-old woman who refused therapy because she had psychologically assimilated her tumor as an essential component of self. The mass measured approximately 15 cm in diameter and was protected by tensely attenuated skin which transmitted a labyrinth of dilated blood vessels (Fig. 7-15). A needle aspirate demonstrated a fibrillar, blue, almost waxy matrix in which polyhedral epithelial cells and dendritic or fusiform chondroid elements coexisted (Fig. 7-16). These mesenchymal cells in a milieu of fibrillar ground substance in association with epithelial cells containing delicate nuclear membranes and eccentrically-situated nucleoli are features ascribed to mixed tumors or pleomorphic adenomas.[6] The latter term is preferred because of the postulated purely epithelial genesis of these tumors. When the mass was ultimately excised, the transected surface appeared lobulated, variegated, hemorrhagic and irregularly gelatinous (Fig. 7-17). The histology characterized the union of the epithelial stellate and trabecular aggregates in a cartilaginous-like stroma (Fig. 7-18). The absence of infiltrative, destructive growth and its projected cellular atypia allowed assignment to a benign classification commensurate with slow progression over many years. The pleomorphic adenoma is the most common parotid neoplasm in our aspirate series. A second fascinating lesion with which we have had recur-

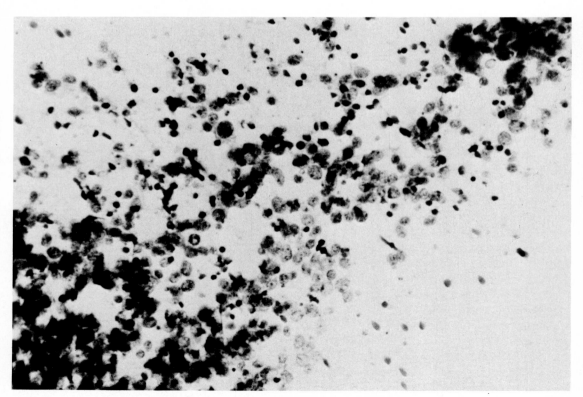

Fig. 7-11. Papanicolaou stain, 400×, fine needle aspirate, metastatic small cell undifferentiated carcinoma.

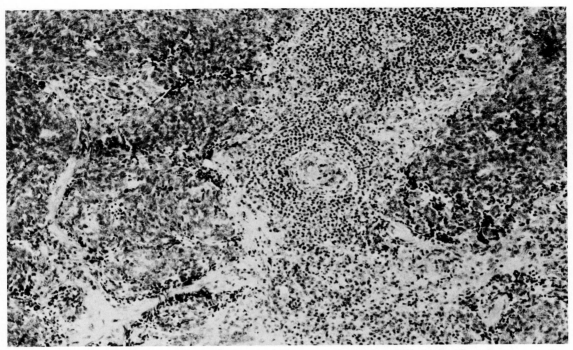

Fig. 7-12. Histologic section, H&E, 160×, metastatic small cell undifferentiated carcinoma.

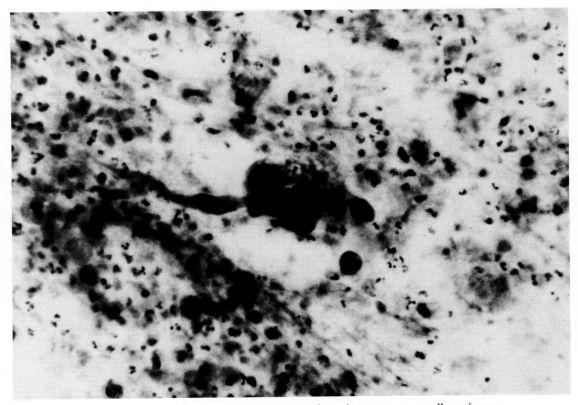

Fig. 7-13. Papanicolaou stain, 400×, metastatic cavitary squamous cell carcinoma.

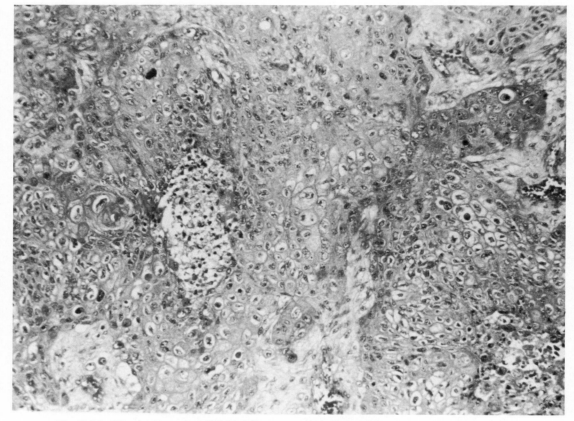

Fig. 7-14. Histologic section, H&E, 160×, metastatic keratinizing squamous cell carcinoma.

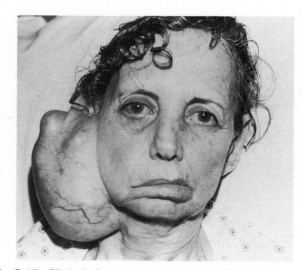

Fig. 7-15. Clinical photograph, pleomorphic adenoma of parotid.

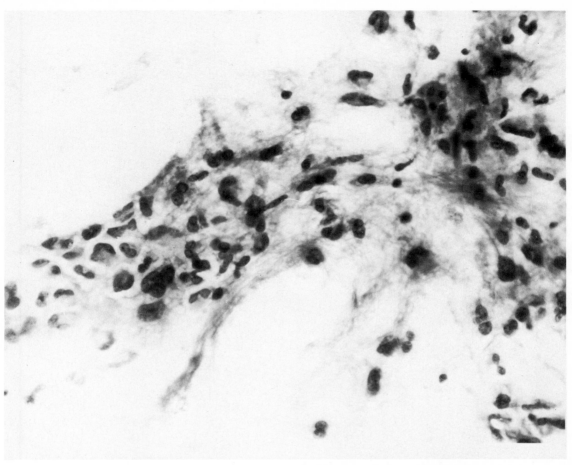

Fig. 7-16. Papanicolaou stain, 400×, needle aspirate, pleomorphic adenoma of parotid.

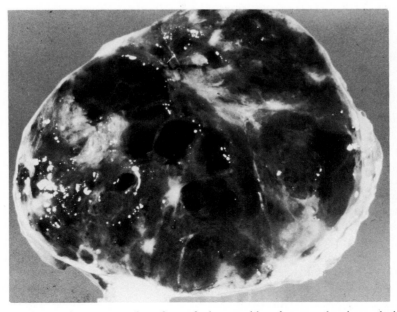

Fig. 7-17. Gross specimen, the transected surface of pleomorphic adenoma showing gelatinous lobulation, hemorrhage, and cystic degeneration.

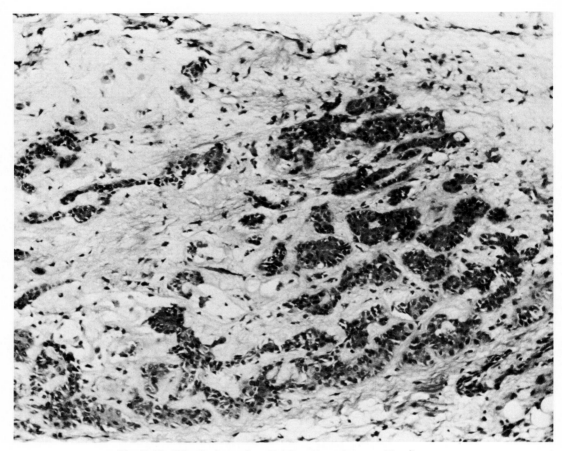

Fig. 7-18. Histologic section, H&E, 160×, pleomorphic adenoma.

rent exposure is represented by an aspirate from a 3-cm, well-delineated, thinly encapsulated, partially cystic mass at the edge of parotid parenchyma in a 68-year-old man (Fig. 7-19). The tumor provided a cellular population consisting of large aggregates of columnar cells with well-delimited cytoplasmic margins and pronounced eosinophilia surrounded by diffusely disported lymphocytes (Fig. 7-20). The former are considered to represent oncocytes which are characterized by their distinct cytoplasmic outlines, eosinophilia and high degree of cellular cohesion.[5] These cells are requisite to classification of this lesion appropriately as papillary cystadenoma lymphomatosum, but when they are observed in preponderant proportions exempt from a lymphocytic population, oncocytoma must be considered. The histological pattern is clearly unique and consists of cystic

spaces invaginated by lymphoid stroma supporting palisaded oncocytic cells with regimentation in perfect alignment (Fig. 7-21). Eneroth and Zajicek[5] emphasized that recognition of oncocytes in smears with cyst fluid and lymphocytes has improved their diagnostic accuracy from 24% in 1953–1962 to 83% in 1963–1964.

The potential of fine needle aspiration cytology in the evaluation of salivary gland lesions may be exercised to provide information relating directly to the preoperative recognition of tumor, formulation of the operative plan to encompass limited resection or wide, radical excision, and decisions to prescribe preoperative or primary irradiation. In the Scandinavian studies[4,7] the preoperative recognition of the lesions *as tumors* was achieved in 92% of the cases. The remaining 8% were classified as "false negatives" but, actually represented unsuitable acellular speci-

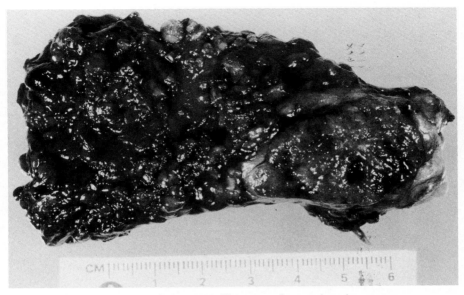

Fig. 7-19. Gross specimen, papillary cystadenoma lymphomatosum.

mens derived from tumors with cystic degeneration, particularly mucoepidermoid carcinomas.[8] Evacuation of fluid eventuating in resolution of a palpatory mass could justify assignment of the patient to a medical surveillance program, but persistence of induration constituted reason for biopsy. Statistics generated in this series essentially disregarded the possibility of false positives. In a compilation of 274 cases of benign tumor, a false positive diagnosis of malignancy occurred in only one instance.[4] The cytological characteristics could reliably project the histoarchitecture in more than 80% of cases. A limitation is apparently imposed when the tumor is malignant because the cytological preparation does not reliably establish this potential in more than 25% of cases. The acceptability of this information is augmented by the relatively inconsequential risk of biopsy, which does not threaten hemorrhage, infection, or seeding of tumor along the needle tract. The latter consideration was studied in seven benign resections of encapsulated masses, and no tumor was discovered beyond the capsule. There were no recurrences in 89 cases observed for 5 years postoperatively despite antecedent needle aspiration. With time and confidence, this technique will offer comfort, familiarity, reliability, and rapid diagnosis of salivary gland lesions.

SUSPICIOUS LYMPH NODES

Alien epithelial cells that molest a lymph node can be readily distinguished from the fundamental hematopoietic population in fine needle aspirates of lymphadenopathy, and may be compared to the source for verification of structure.[12] Investigation of lymph nodes by this technique is predicated on the impetus to search for metastatic carcinoma. The procedure has not been considered satisfactory for the primary diagnosis of malignant lymphomas.[10] Lymph nodes were the most frequently aspirated structure in Frable's initial series[9] and the amended report.[10] Head and neck cancers were the most frequent primary sites and squamous cell carcinoma dominated the histoarchitectural pattern of the source lesion. Of the nodes aspirated in the head and neck, 79% had associated primary tumors above and 21% below the diaphragm. This distribution, however, is at variance with the report from the Karolinska Institute,[12] although it conforms to other experiences. Frable's head and neck study incorporated 567 biopsies of which 323 were lymph nodes. Of these, 171 contained metastatic carcinoma cells. The aspirated nodes were distributed primarliy in the anterior cervical chain (199 cases), then in the supraclavicular region (81 cases), and less frequently in the

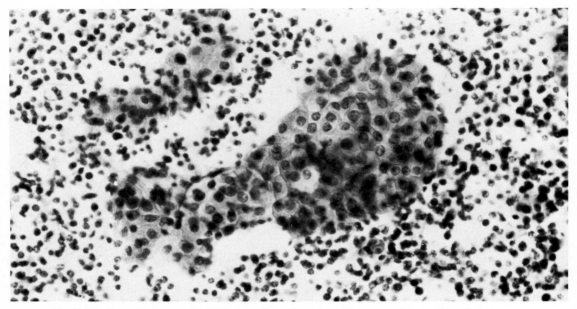

Fig. 7-20. Papanicolaou stain, 200×, needle aspirate, papillary cystadenoma lymphomatosum.

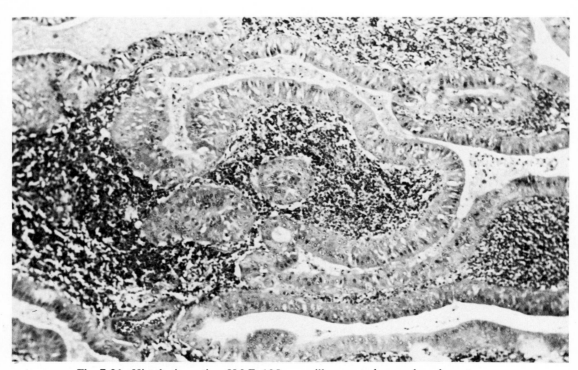

Fig. 7-21. Histologic section, H&E, 125×, papillary cystadenoma lymphomatosum.

submaxillary or submandibular zone (36 cases). The supraclavicular deposits were generally from sites other than head and neck, usually lung and breast. The Memorial Hospital study[11] reported malignant cells in 125 of 220 lymph node aspirates, and all were confirmed by subsequent tissue examination. The technique may improve the accuracy of lymphangiography.[13] In our own developing but limited experience, metastatic carcinoma is the most commonly reported diagnostic result of aspiration biopsy of lymph nodes because we actively discourage the technique for investigating enlarged nodes clinically suspected to be manifestations of Hodgkin's disease or other lymphomas.

Our most commonly identified tumors are squamous cell carcinomas, adenocarcinomas, malignant melanomas, and undifferentiated cancers. Figure 7-22 demonstrates polyhedral and spindle cells with keratinizing cytoplasm and homogenized, hyperchromatic nuclei derived from an enlarged node replaced by grey-white, friable tumor (Fig. 7-23). Histologically, the characteristic mosaic of squamous carcinoma is reproduced in an alien environment at the expense of nodal architecture (Figure 7-24).

Glandular constructions are obviously loyal to acinar patterns with preservation of prominent nucleoli, delicately vacuolated cytoplasm and pseudopapillary affiliations (Figures 7-25, 7-26). The availability of the tissue provides a medium for observing the cells in arbitrary sheets or reviewing their features with applications of mucicarmine stains (Fig. 7-27).

Frable reported lymphadenitis, reactive hyperplasia or a related phenomenon in 116 of his lymph node cases and relied on a mixed cellular pattern of comingled stimulated lymphocytes of variable size, plasma cells and histiocytes with phagocytosis to decide that the process was benign. This was useful to us in our analyses, and benign processes declared from slide reviews of aspiration biopsies were confirmed with time and clinical resolution. The ability of the technique to offer this distinction is suggested by the study case we include here for illustration. A 66-year-old male presented with axillary and inguinal lymphadenopathy of 3 month's duration (Fig. 7-28). Needle aspirates from both regions contained a mixed population of lymphohistiocytic elements with multinucleated giant cells (Figs. 7-29 and 7-30). A diagnosis of granuloma-

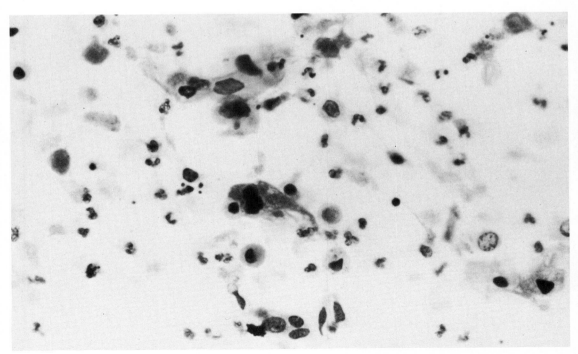

Fig. 7-22. Papanicolaou stain, 625×, needle aspirate, metastatic squamous cell carcinoma.

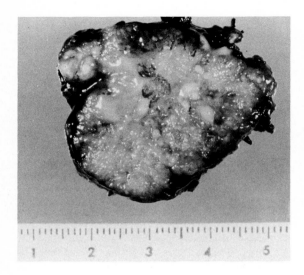

Fig. 7-23. Gross specimen, excised lymph node with metastatic squamous cell carcinoma.

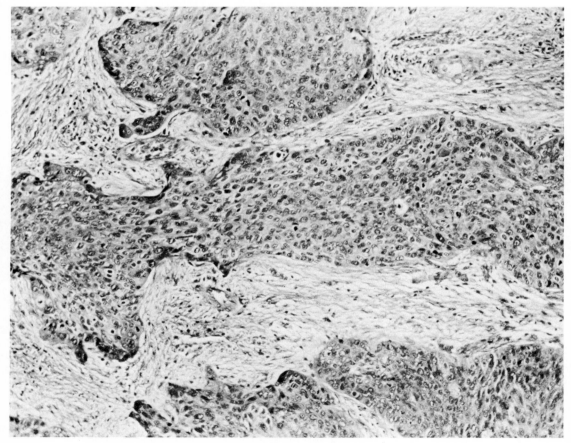

Fig. 7-24. Histologic section, H&E, 160×, metastatic squamous cell carcinoma.

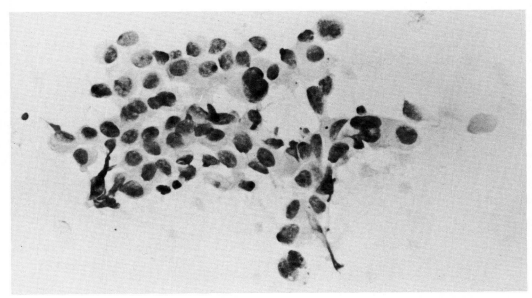

Fig. 7-25. Papanicolaou stain, 400×, needle aspirate, metastatic adenocarcinoma.

tous lymphadenitis prompted open biopsy for confirmation and to obtain tissue for acid fast and fungal cultures. The node was extensively effaced by a reactive process that provided multinucleated histiocytes but no evidence for caseation necrosis (Fig. 7-31). A peculiar variant was the occurrence of rod-shaped, homogenized, refractile, eosinophilic crystalline deposits demonstrated to consist of precipitated immunoglobulins (Fig. 7-32).

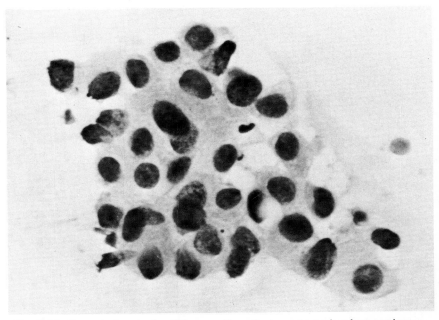

Fig. 7-26. Papanicolaou stain, 625×, needle aspirate, metastatic adenocarcinoma.

Frable used the presence of empty vacuoles within lymphocyte nuclei coupled with the absence of phagocytosis to predict a lymphoma from thin needle aspirates of clinically enlarged lymph nodes. He cautioned that identification may be possible for a virgin diagnosis, but that classification should not be attempted, except to distinguish between Hodgkin's and non-Hodgkin's lymphoma. He emphasized that the "usefulness of aspiration biopsy in the diagnosis of lymphoma lies in proving the involvement of node groups that appear clinically suspicious, demonstrating recurrence or extension to new groups of lymph nodes after or during therapy, and separating lymphomas from lymphadenitis." Figure 7-33 demonstrates the pure lymphoid population retrieved intraoperatively from an enlarged submaxillary node in a 6-year-old female. The monomorphous population of lymphocytes with prominent, often multiple nucleoli lead to a diagnosis of lymphoma, but classification was deferred until the entire node was excised. The tumor proved to be a Burkitt's lymphoma (Fig. 7-34) without jaw involvement (Fig. 7-35), but this process, ironically, incorporates phagocytosis as a characteristic that is generally reserved for benign lymphadenitis. This may eventuate in entrapment, misjudgment and inappropriate patient management. The caveat cannot be too strongly stressed that aspiration cytology is limited as a technique for diagnosis and classification of malignant lymphoma. The blatant exception is the demonstration of unequivocal Dorothy Reed Sternberg cells in nodal aspirates from patients with classical evidence for Hodgkin's disease.

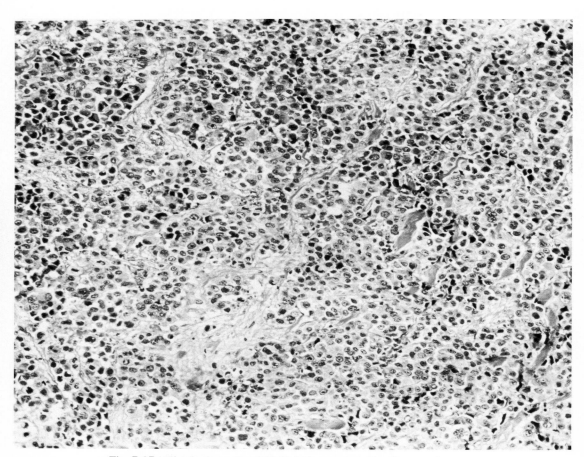

Fig. 7-27. Histologic section, H&E, 160×, metastatic adenocarcinoma.

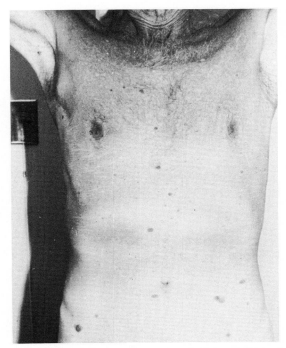

Fig. 7-28. Clinical photograph, axillary and inguinal lymphadenopathy.

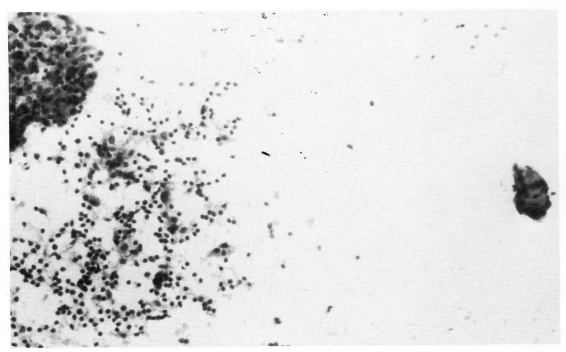

Fig. 7-29. Papanicolaou stain, 400×, needle aspirate, granulomatous lymphadenitis.

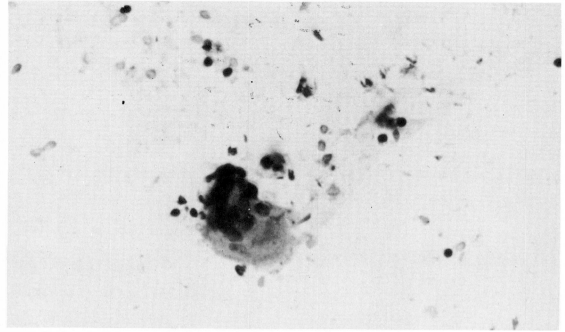

Fig. 7-30. Papanicolaou stain, 400×, needle aspirate, multinucleated giant cell of granulomatous lymphadenitis.

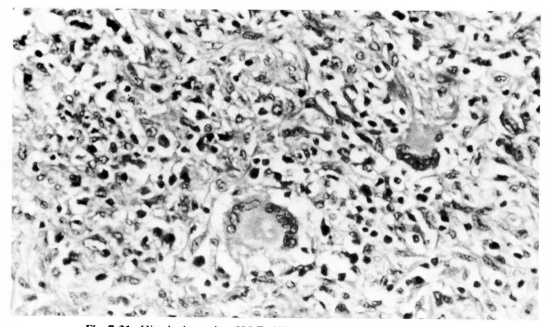

Fig. 7-31. Histologic section, H&E, 400×, granulomatous lymphadenitis.

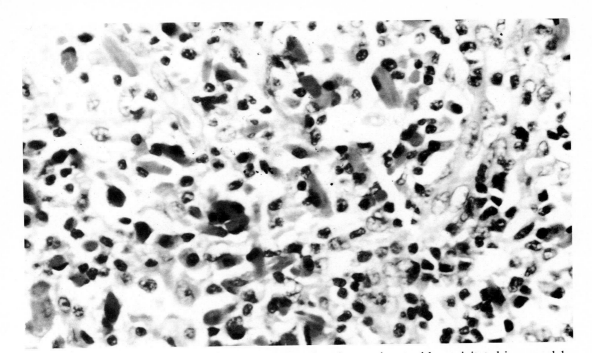

Fig. 7-32. Histologic section, H&E, 400×, rectangular deposits, consistent with precipitated immunoglobulins.

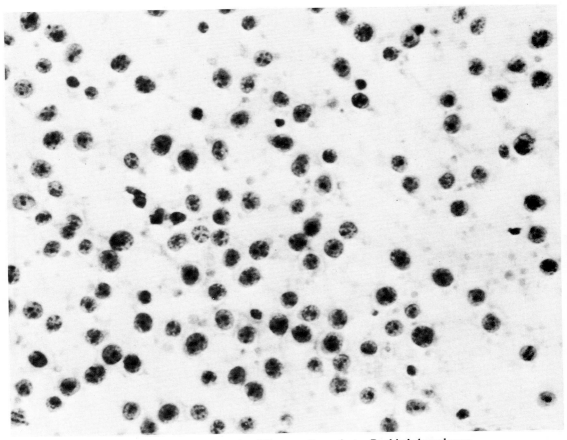

Fig. 7-33. Papanicolaou stain, 625×, needle aspirate, Burkitt's lymphoma.

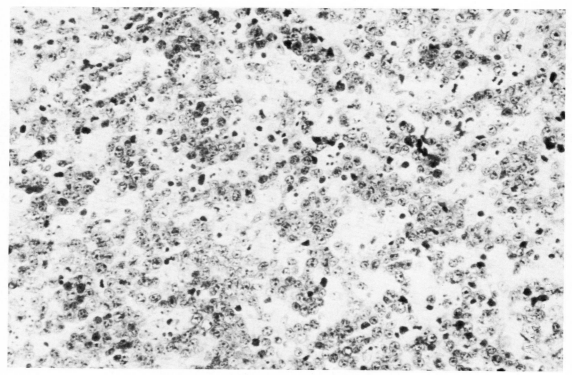

Fig. 7-34. Histologic section, H&E, 400×, Burkitt's lymphoma.

ACCESSIBLE BONE LESIONS

Fluoroscopy, radionuclide imaging techniques, and direct palpation may guide the needle to a suspicious or destructive bone lesion to acquire cells for substantiation of a metastatic carcinoma or a primary bone tumor. The reported experience implies a reticence to use the technique in deference to the consensus that interpretation of even histologic material requires an intensive collaborative effort with correlation of radiographs, clinical presentation, age, and location to ensure an enlightened collective opinion before mutilating surgery, radiation, or systemic chemotherapy are prescribed. In Frable's small series[9] metastatic tumors equally divided between breast and lung cancers were the most commonly aspirated lesions of bone. Hajdu and Melamed[11] reported 37 of 39 bone aspirates as metastatic epidermoid or adenocarcinoma. A detailed morphologic diagnosis was possible for 31 of 46 lesions suspected to be primary bone tumors and for 39 of 48 cases of

postulated metastatic tumors in Stormby and Akerman's[14] series. They advocated the technique as an early adjunct to histologic diagnosis rather than a substitute for it, citing caveats to interpretation such as the ubiquitous occurrence of giant cells, which are difficult to assess when dissociated from tissue organization. Akerman[15] subsequently reassured that the reliability of needle aspiration of bone was 90%.

The primary diagnosis and management of bone tumors is an infrequent occurrence in the community hospital, and convention usually predicts a course of open biopsy with histologic study rather than early, direct confrontation by needle aspiration. This may be somewhat less valid for examination of the suspected metastatic lesion. Both account for the paucity of material in the medium of aspiration cytology, and the restriction of illustrative examples: A 6-year-old male presented with a pathologic fracture of the femur. A preliminary x-ray demonstrated a destructive mass with periosteal elevation and extension (Fig. 7-36). Aspirates demonstrated

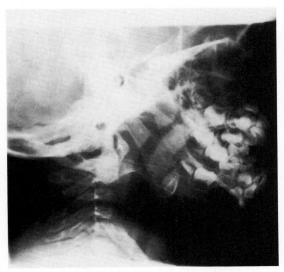

Fig. 7-35. Clinical x-ray demonstrating the absence of tumor in the patient's jaw.

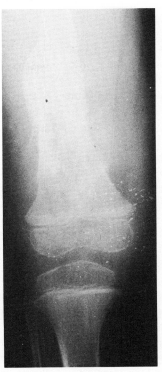

Fig. 7-36. Clinical x-ray, femoral mass and Codman's triangle of osteogenic sarcoma.

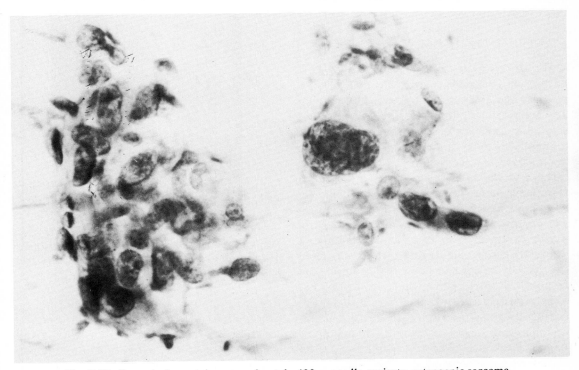

Fig. 7-37. Papanicolaou stain, approximately 400×, needle aspirate, osteogenic sarcoma.

large, pleomorphic cells with coarsely precipitated chromatin, associated with aggregates of smaller mesenchymal cells (Fig. 7-37). Eosinophilic, homogenized amorphous deposits were occasionally seen adjacent to cells or in the background detritus and represented osteoid particles. The disarticulated leg contributed the femur ravaged by aggressive tumor, which destroyed the cortex in its periosteal avalanche (Fig. 7-38). Decalcified sections demonstrated proliferating malignant osteoblasts with trabecular deposition of osteoid and marginal, haphazard alignment of the offending cells (Fig. 7-39). A 66-year-old male with prostatic adenocarcinoma (Fig. 7-42) and elevated acid phosphatase presented with multifocal bone pain. A radionuclide bone search disclosed multiple areas of increased activity consistent with disseminated carcinoma (Fig. 7-40). An aspirate from the iliac crest without local anesthesia or subsequent complication harvested epithelial cells in a glandular pattern correlative with the primary tumor (Fig. 7-41). This is an extreme case with heavy presumptive evidence for metastatic spread, but serves to reinforce the availability of a technique which can replace assumption with certainty.

CONCLUDING REMARKS

We are privileged to practice cytopathology in an era of medical achievement that dictates progress and excellence in the diagnostic method. Sophisticated adjunctive techniques have evolved to augment the histologic evaluation of tumors. Scanning and transmission electron microscopy, surface markers, immunofluorescence, and chemical determinants of hormonal responsiveness amplify the armamentarium. Yet these advanced techniques are time-consuming and expensive, complicating escalating costs of health care and delaying the information of cancer diagnosis and staging for the apprehensive patient anxious to know of his status and prognosis. It is refreshing that a technique has been reintroduced, which allows a definitive bedside diagnosis that may frequently circumvent surgical biopsy or lengthy radiographic staging procedures, and concomitantly restrict costs while providing a rapid analysis. Aspiration

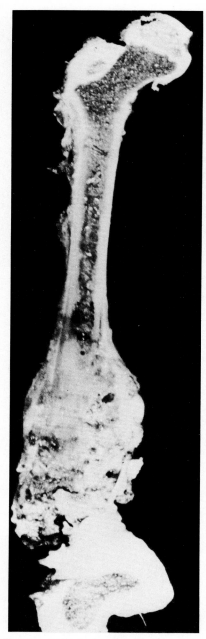

Fig. 7-38. Femur from disarticulated lower extremity demonstrating destructive proliferation of osteogenic sarcoma.

biopsy offers the community hospital a precise, cost-effective, rapid primary diagnostic modality whose ramifications portend a revolutionary influence on the diagnostic effort, by deter-

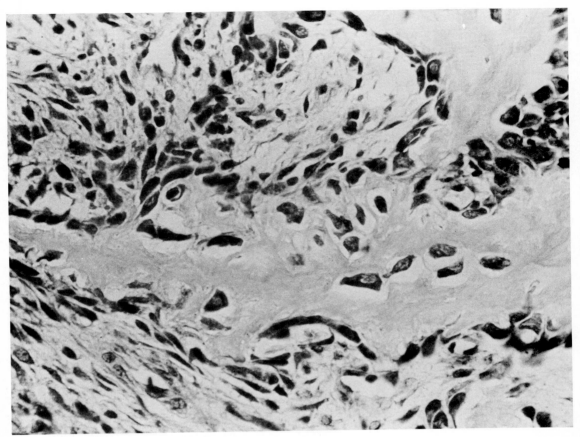

Fig. 7-39. Histologic section, H&E, approximately 200×, osteogenic sarcoma.

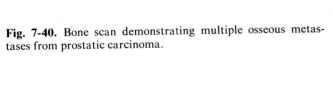

Fig. 7-40. Bone scan demonstrating multiple osseous metastases from prostatic carcinoma.

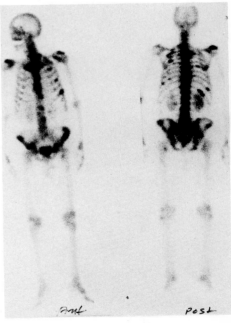

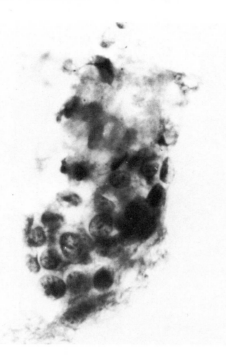

Fig. 7-41. Papanicolaou stain, 625×, needle aspirate, metastatic adenocarcinoma, consistent with origin from prostatic primary.

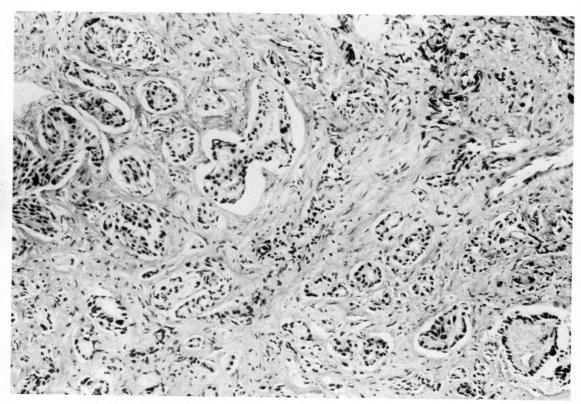

Fig. 7-42. Histologic section, H&E, 160×, primary adenocarcinoma of prostate.

mining a trend for enthusiastic, considerate, and cost-conscious responsibility in the delivery of health care.

REFERENCES

1. Hajdu, S. I., and Hajdu, E. O.: *Cytopathology of Sarcomas and Other Nonepithelial Malignant Tumors.* W. B. Saunders Co., Philadelphia, 1976.
2. Akerman, M., Idvall, I., and Rydholm, A.: Cytodiagnosis of soft tissue tumors and tumor-like conditions by means of fine needle aspiration biopsy. *Arch Orthop Traum Surg* **96:** 61–67, 1980.
3. Kline, T. A., Neal, H. S., and Holroyde, C. P.: Needle Aspiration Biopsy, Diagnosis of Subcutaneous Nodules and Lymph Nodes. *JAMA* **235:** 2848–2850, 1976.
4. Mavec, P., Eneroth, C. M., Franzen, S., Moberger, G., and Zajicek, J.: Aspiration Biopsy of Salivary Gland Tumors, I. Correlation of Cytologic Reports from 652 Aspiration Biopsies with Clinical and Histologic Findings. *Acta Otolaryng* **58:** 471–484, 1964.
5. Eneroth, C. M., and Zajicek, J.: Aspiration biopsy of salivary gland tumors. II. Morphologic studies on smears and histologic sections from oncocytic tumors (45 cases of papillary cystadenoma lymphomatosum and 4 cases of oncocytoma). *Acta Cytologica* **9**(5): 355–361, 1965.
6. Eneroth, C. M., and Zajicek, J.: Aspiration biopsy of salivary gland tumors. III. Morphologic studies on smears and histologic sections from 368 mixed tumors. *Acta Cytologica* **10**(6): 440–454, 1966.
7. Eneroth, C. M., Franzen, S., and Zajicek, J.: Aspiration biopsy of salivary gland tumors. A critical review of 910 biopsies. *Acta Cytologica* **11**(5): 470–472, 1967.
8. Lindberg, L. G., and Akerman, M.: Aspiration cytology of salivary gland tumors: Diagnostic experience from six years of routine laboratory work. *Laryngoscope.* **86**(4): 584–594, 1976.
9. Frable, W. J.: Thin-needle aspiration biopsy. A personal experience with 469 cases. *Am J Clin Pathol* **65**(2): 168–182, 1976.
10. Frable, W. J., and Frable, M. A.: Thin-needle aspiration biopsy. The diagnosis of head and neck tumors revisited. *Cancer* **43**(4): 1541–1548, 1979.
11. Hajdu, S. I., and Melamed, M. R.: The diagnostic value of aspiration smears. *Am J Clin Pathol* **59**(3): 350–356, 1973.
12. Engzell, U., Jakobsson, P. A., Sigurdson, A., and Zajicek, J.: Aspiration biopsy of metastatic carcinoma in lymph nodes of the neck. *Acta Otolaryng* **72:** 138–174, 1971.
13. Thomson, K. R., House, A. J. S., Gothlin, J. H., and Dolan, T. E.: Percutaneous lymph node aspiration biopsy: Experience with a new technique. *Clin Radiol* **28:** 329–332, 1977.
14. Stormby, N. and Akerman, Mans: Cytodiagnosis of bone lesions by means of fine-needle aspiration biopsy. *Acta Cytol* **17:** 166–172, 1973.
15. Akerman, M., Berg, N. O., and Persson, B. M.: Fine needle aspiration biopsy in the evaluation of tumor-like lesions of bone. *Acta Orthop Scand* **47:** 129–136, 1976.

Index

Page numbers in *italics* indicate illustrations or diagrams